Creative Play & Drama

with Adults at Risk

Creative Play & Drama

with Adults at Risk

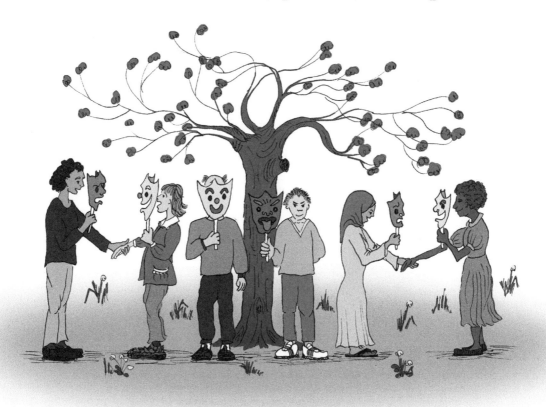

Sue Jennings

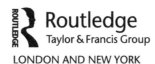
Routledge
Taylor & Francis Group

LONDON AND NEW YORK

I would like to dedicate this book to Roger Grainger, who more than anyone else has written, reserched and performed drama and theatre work and dramatherapy for so many groups of people at risk.

Cover picture and illustrations by Chloe Gerhardt

Drawings for Worksheets 3.1, 5.3, 5.4 and 8.5 by Suzanne Hall

Thank you both.

First published 2003 by Speechmark Publishing Ltd.

Published 2017 by Routledge
2 Park Square, Milton Park, Abingdon, Oxon OX14 4RN
711 Third Avenue, New York, NY 10017, USA

Routledge is an imprint of the Taylor & Francis Group, an informa business

British Library Cataloguing in Publication Data
Jennings, Sue, 1938–
     Creative play and drama with adults at risk. - (A Speechmark therapy resource)
     1. Psychodrama 2. Drama – Therapeutic use   3. Recreational therapy
     I. Title
     616.8'91523

ISBN: 9780863885358 (pbk)

Contents

List of Worksheets

Acknowledgements

I WISH TO THANK Sandy Ackerman and Dave Evans for being such creative drama colleagues, especially in the field of peer education and social theatre. I deeply miss the late Clive Barker who died before I had finished this book, who has always been a profound influence on my work.

Everyone at Speechmark, especially Miranda Robson, gives me unfailing support. Suzannne Hall has typed and proofread in her excellent way. Family and friends have been tolerant as I completed the fourth volume of these creative approaches to my work.

Introduction

WE ARE ALL INFLUENCED BY our earliest roots, and there is no doubt that my childhood experience as a dancer and community performer led me to theatre school and has continued to contribute to my world view. As a student, I was invited to work in the local psychiatric hospital – 'doing drama' on the ward.

Background and Perspectives

My academic background is in theatre studies, social anthropology and eco-studies and sustainability. My doctoral fieldwork, 'Theatre, Ritual and Transformation', took place in the Malaysian rainforest with a tribal people, the Senoi Temiar, where I was studying ritual and performance.

My working life continues to include:

- The application of theatre and dramatherapy in areas of 'special need', preferably working within a team that includes the institution's staff.
- Work with people as varied as those seeking fertility treatment, serial killers in maximum security institutions, children and adults with learning difficulties, nuns in a convent, mothers and babies, people with personality disorders.
- Continuing development of appropriate training in cross-cultural contexts both for specialists and institutional staff, especially in eastern Europe.
- The maintenance of my own sanity through acting in the theatre.
- The recording of all these experiences in books and articles and allowing them to grow in an organic way.

Theoretical Influences on My Work

Shakespeare

His theatre and plays

> a fiction … a dream of passion
> (*Hamlet* 2, ii)

> abstract and brief chronicles of time
> (*Hamlet* 2, ii)

> I could a tale unfold whose lightest word
> Would harrow up thy soul
> (*Hamlet* 1, v)

> This wide and universal theatre
> Presents more woeful pageants than the scene
> Wherein we play in.
> (*As You Like It* 2, vii)

His meticulous observation and perception of the effects of theatre

> The play's the thing
> Wherein I'll catch the conscience of the king
> (*Hamlet* 2, ii)

> Condemn the fault and not the actor of it?
> (*Measure for Measure* 2, ii)

> ... so you shall hear
> Of carnal, bloody, and unnatural acts,
> Of accidental judgements, casual slaughters,
> Of deaths put on by cunning and false cause
> (*Hamlet* 5, ii)

> A showing of a heavenly effect in an earthly actor
> (*All's Well That Ends Well* 2, iii)

Theorists Who Have Written About the Theatre

- Antonin Artaud and his political stance on mental illness and his search for a new, 'visceral' language of theatre (Artaud, 1958).
- Peter Slade and 'Child Drama'.
- Dorothy Heathcote and 'Drama-in-Education'.
- Vygotsky's theories of learning through social interaction and through language: his 'scaffolding' approach to developmental learning (Vygotsky 1978).
- Brecht's concept of alienation and Brook's 're-presentation'.
- Wilshire and 'mimetic involvement' and 'embodied experience' (Wilshire, 1982).
- The work of Turner (1982), Schechner (1985, 1991), Boal (1992), Lewis, Tambiah.

New Developments in Neuroscience

- Cozolino and the contribution of arts and play to the repair of damaged neurons and re-building of the brain (Cozolino, 2002).
- Narrative theory and analysis – co-constructed and performed narratives.
- Systemic theory, Bateson, Bronfenbrenner, including the 'eco-system' of gender – Bandura 'social learning theory'.

- Recent writings on social theatre and applied theatre: Schinina (2004), Somers, Taylor (2003), Thompson (1994).

In this Book

Chapter 1: So What is this Drama Stuff? looks at the many words for describing drama work in the context of people with 'special needs' and places it in a historical context. The emergence of psychodrama and dramatherapy are placed within the broad spectrum of the therapeutic field. The title of this chapter arises from a question asked of me by the Finance Department when I arrived to work at a new hospital!

Chapter 2: The Play of Life and the Drama of Life looks at the developmental model of drama (EPR) – Embodiment–Projection–Role – and its adaptability. It also looks at the groups of people who can benefit from drama and dramatherapy, and some of the outcomes of this approach to creative work.

Chapter 3: Ancient Wisdom for Changing Times describes the importance of old stories and plays, and there are many exercises to develop drama work on texts of different kinds.

Chapter 4: Games, Games and Yet More Games discusses several types of games and their role in the drama group, including games that are used for warm-ups, 'set games' and status games. Psychological game-playing is also discussed, especially in relation to bullying.

Chapter 5: A Little Touch of Something emphasises the importance of touch and the senses, but is placed sensitively within the context of the abuse that many people have suffered.

Chapter 6: A Voice for All Seasons describes how we can develop our voices both for promoting health as well as building confidence. Various breathing and voice techniques are described.

Chapter 7: Bring on the Clowns introduces the theme of humour and how clowns play an important part in our overall creative development. There are many clowning techniques and warm-ups.

Chapter 8: Creative Playing between Adults and Children looks at the stages of play and how children can help adults learn to play again. The use of improvisation and the development of the imagination are described, together with a wide range of techniques.

Chapter 9: Drama Techniques and Strategies is about how we organise our drama workshops and the physical, psychological, spiritual and social benefits of doing drama. The importance of creativity and artistry is developed for all our groups.

Chapter 10: Play, Theatre and Performance takes us into the culmination of this work, which emphasises the importance of performance, especially through Shakespearean texts and tales. Masks are included as a final dimension to the creative drama work.

Chapter 11: Resources provides useful addresses for information and training.

Chapter 12: Bibliography includes both books cited in the text and suggested useful reading.

Sue Jennings
Somerset 2005

CHAPTER 1

So What is this Drama Stuff?

> ...so surprised my sense
> That I was nothing.
> (Shakespeare, *The Winter's Tale* 3, i, 10)

> What do you read, my lord? – Words, words, words.
> (Shakespeare, *Hamlet* 2, ii, 194)

THE LAST CENTURY CREATED A PANOPLY of words with which people tried to describe drama and theatre in practice, such as:

- Theatre-in-education
- Applied theatre
- Drama-in-education
- Drama therapy (US)
- Therapeutic theatre
- Social drama
- Psychodrama
- ritual theatre
- Para-theatre
- Playback theatre
- Performance theatre
- Re-staging
- Child drama
- Healing theatre
- Role play
- Dramatherapy
- Social theatre
- Dramatic play
- Forum theatre
- Enactment
- Action method
- Developmental theatre
- Theatre of the oppressed
- Theatre therapy
- Remedial drama
- Theatre of sources
- Drama in therapy

The last century also saw the rise and further rise of the status of psychology and various forms of psychological theories and therapies; thus we have, for example:

- Psychoanalysis
- Psychotherapy
- Psychosynthesis
- Analytic psychotherapy
- Group psychotherapy
- Child psychology
- Counselling psychology
- Couple (formerly marital) psychotherapy
- Cognitive analytic therapy

- Educational psychology
- Cognitive-behavioural therapy
- Neuropsychology
- Social psychology
- Applied psychology
- Developmental psychology
- Child psychoanalysis
- Clinical psychology
- Humanistic psychology

Where is the hapless arts worker to stand in all this? Since the State Registration of dramatherapists (and other arts therapists), practitioners are a little nervous: are they attempting to 'do' dramatherapy? Provided that it is not named as such, is that all right? Because with State Registration comes 'protection of title' and now no-one can use the title 'dramatherapist' or refer to what they do as 'dramatherapy', unless they have followed an approved course and are on the register of the Health Professions Council (HPC). We have to call what we do something else! Hence my idea for the title of this book: *Creative Play and Drama with Adults at Risk*.

However, I think it is useful for us to consider a little of the background of 'play, drama and theatre with special populations', before we go further into our journey through this book. Some of the initiatives turned into therapies, others stayed as creative drama and theatre developments. None of the initiatives have had a smooth passage!

Dramatherapy and Psychodrama

Beginnings

The first half of the twentieth century saw one of the early attempts to make psychological therapy more active through the work of psychiatrist Jacob Moreno. Moreno, who was Romanian by birth, finally settled in the USA and developed there his theory and practice of psychodrama. Moreno experimented with spontaneous theatre with children and adults, telling stories and incorporating dramatic methods into his fledgling practice. He worked with professional actors in his own theatre, and created a public theatre space where people could enact their difficulties in the 'here and now' and consider strategies for change.

Catharsis has always been an important aspect of psychodramatic work, and over the years Moreno established a core of techniques based on role-play, and a working structure for group work. This formed the basis for the psychodrama movement, with formalised training which started in the US and travelled to the UK.

> The locus of psychodrama, if necessary, may be designed everywhere, wherever the patients are, the field of battle, the classroom or the private home. But the ultimate resolution of deep mental conflicts requires an objective setting, the therapeutic theatre.
> (Moreno, 1934)

Within the same time frame, dramatherapy seems to have started on both sides of the ocean with expressive drama classes, creative dramatics and drama games with drama and theatre specialists (Casson, 2004), and post-war play readings in occupational therapy activities. However, it seemed there was no one inspired individual until Peter Slade achieved a milestone when he put the two words drama and therapy together (1959). Slade applied his principles, which he had developed in *Child Drama* (1954) to his therapeutic work, with groups of people with special needs, whether in hospitals, prisons or schools. Slade emphasises the importance of drama and dramatic play in a child's early years, without it leading to formal performance:

> There was no stage just space; no audience, no axe to grind, no money to be made, no grown-up to titter to disturb the acting, no showing off, no worries, no clapping, nothing done for propaganda, it was not a social event. It was all done for the right reason. We were absorbed in creating real Child Drama, because we loved it and because we felt (we actually *experienced*) that we were creating something wonderful and beautiful.
> (Slade, 1995).

These early beginnings of expressive drama and drama games in dramatherapy, and spontaneous theatre in psychodrama are both characterised by their roots in theatre arts, though interestingly enough there seems to have been little knowledge at the time of the experimental theatre work of Stanislavski and his influence in the traditional theatre of his day.

The Victorians also built theatres in their large psychiatric institutions where patients and staff could be entertained, and where patients themselves would occasionally perform. There then seems to have been a gradual erosion of any major reference to theatre as such. It is the dramatic action that becomes the focus through which people address issues in their lives and children can become more confident and creative. Slade is very clear that there is no audience and no stage and although Moreno staged his own work in theatres with an audience, he later went on to say that his main task was to break down the barriers between actors and audience.

Issues of performance, artistry and aesthetics were slowly supplanted by action, feelings, and real life. Apart from the work of a few charismatic practitioners, drama as a creative process and an action method became separated from the context of theatre. The only variations arose from a few individual initiatives. For example, Elsie Green, a theatre director who worked from 1952 to 1984 at Horton Psychiatric Hospital in Surrey, UK, was unknown to the UK and US dramatherapy field until her biography (Walton, 1998) was reviewed in *The Prompt* (Casson, 2001). Green proved to be one of the few theatre-based people to continue work in therapy, and indeed describes her practice as 'theatre therapy' (Walton, 1998).

Dramatherapy and Psychodrama Today

Both dramatherapy and psychodrama now share the decrease of specific theatre structure and technique in their practice. However there are still some major differences between dramatherapy and psychodrama that were apparent at the outset. For example, psychodrama works through an individual protagonist (see also Chesner, 1994), and the difficulties of the individual are seen to be the difficulties of the whole group. In dramatherapy the focus is on the collaboration of the group as a whole, where issues can be addressed indirectly through creative drama and expression (Watts, 1992).

Since the 1960s, dramatherapy, psychodrama and other new action approaches have proliferated through parallel processes in health and education in many countries: many initiatives started by individuals developed without knowledge of other peoples' work. Most practitioners saw their work as drama based and placed in a context of either social drama, psychodrama or action work.

During the late 1970s and 1980s there was a major shift from praxis to training: new careers and professions were created, with professional associations that took people in and kept others out. Formalised postgraduate training was established in several universities and private organisations, both for dramatherapy and psychodrama. There were now dramatherapists and psychodramatists looking for work.

The 1990s brought even greater concerns about professionalisation. In the UK, dramatherapists applied to join a national health professions register, now the Health Professions Council (HPC), with even tighter controls. Psychodramatists applied for recognition as psychotherapists by the United

Kingdom Council for Psychotherapy (UKCP). In the US there is a system of licensing in individual states and many practitioners have to be attached to a department of psychology.

Dramatherapy students are not now required to have a theatre background or at least extended experience of theatre. Whereas in the early years of dramatherapy training, some courses insisted on theatre training as a prerequisite, and students would have to wait while gaining experience in classes and theatre groups (Jennings, 1990). It was thought that immersion in the theatre art forms and experience of artistic performance would form a basis for the training of the dramatherapist. Certainly at one time the actors' union Equity (UK) would give grants for members who wished to train as dramatherapists.

Dramatherapy has taken a little longer to complete its journey to becoming a clinical specialism that joins psychodrama as both a profession and a practice. Dramatherapy does not consider itself to be a theatre practice and is only minimally considered as an education. However, it does claim to provide the 'intentional' use of drama techniques for 'symptom relief' and other therapeutic aims (British Association of Dramatherapists, 1998): after intensive lobbying by a small number of vocal dramatherapists, the phrase 'and theatre' was included!

So as dramatherapy moves further away from theatre, where its roots lie, we can also see that theatre itself has transformed radically in recent years and is given even less importance for funding and development.

Theatre: A Poor Player?

Despite ancient theatre legacy, theatre in recent years has grown away from the centre stage of society. I write at a time when there are 17 musicals on London's West End stage, and there are virtually no regional theatres; the few that are left are receiving houses with no resident company. Major theatre companies can no longer expect young actors to sign long-term contracts because other media might draw them away: indeed many young actors refuse to leave their capital cities because of potential work in film and television. Choices are made between a crowd scene in a commercial and a tour with a theatre-in-education company. Community theatre has not convinced the authorities either. Thompson (1994) talks about theatre and drama in prisons as being seen as another leisure activity or a novel way of presenting teaching materials. He quotes Bidinotto (1994) who writes about theatre in prisons being an 'absurd' privilege which may actually increase the level of crime!

Just as many actors and directors do not see dramatherapy as 'real theatre', 'theatre-in-education' is also seen as something you do when you cannot get 'real theatre' work! As theatre itself becomes more and more marginalised and transformed into spectacle or 'soap', it is not surprising that dramatherapists wish to be nearer to the clinic than the theatre. The clinic is certainly nearer the centre of our increasingly 'problem-focused' society.

The Arts and Health: Scientist and Artist

Some clinicians say that theatre specifically, and the arts in general, not only offer solutions to difficulties but also contribute substantially to the maintenance of health (Russell Davis, 1995, Steinberg, 2002). Some scientists and clinicians are interested in dialogue with artists without wishing to merely take over their methods (Jennings, in preparation). Courtney inspires us by saying:

> Although artistic and scientific creativity have long been thought to be similar, there is this decisive difference; scientists focus their work on external phenomena; even a neurobiologist works on someone else's brain. Performing artists – and, I would say, mediators, shamans, and trancers too – work on themselves, trying to induce deep psychophysical transformations either of a temporary or permanent kind.
>
> (Courtney, 1990)

It is assumed that work that performers do on the self at a deep level is not considered personal development in therapeutic terms. Theatre is still 'not real'; it is artifice and lies, it is 'untrue'. We remember its Greek derivative – *hypokritiki* (hypocrite), 'one who plays a part on a stage'. Plato vilified both the person and the nature of the actor and said that the art of acting could be morally damaging. If a person can represent a bad character on the stage then he (*sic*) cannot be a good person. He maintains that tragedy will excite in the audience emotions that should be curbed:

> Then is it really right, to admire when we see him on the stage, a man we ourselves be ashamed to resemble?
> Is it reasonable to feel enjoyment and admiration rather than disgust?
> (Plato, *The Republic*)

However, in order to be a great scientist it is necessary to have a highly developed and creative imagination. The forming of a hypothesis needs an enormous leap of the imagination (Jennings, 1990): first to consider how something might be, and then return to the laboratory to prove it. Similarly in our creative drama work we encourage children and young people to have flights of fantasy and invention and to take leaps into the unknown although in day-to-day life such activities seem to belong more and more to the infant and junior school. The creative imagination belongs as much to science as it does to the arts, and it needs to be stimulated and developed. Our imagination and intuition need plenty of practice. Nevertheless for Plato the creation of images is the lowest level of mental functioning and art is an avoidance of reality.

The recent research of neuroscientists suggests that play and the arts can have a crucial role in the development of the brain and its functions, and that they might even have a part to play in neuron repair (Cozolino, 2002, Gerhardt, 2004). It is ironic that the scientists are working with theatre artists and not the dramatherapists and play therapists in considering these new ideas!

Theatre and Ritual

Ritual is a spiritual enactment of beliefs and values, or a ritualisation (Turner, 1982) of an important narrative in symbolic terms. Ritual deals with the known factors in our lives in ways that stimulate all our senses and heighten our perception: through incense, food, music, icons and dance. Again, it is a group and social activity. We participate in rituals together and share a common set of values, and most of the time we know what to do: for example if we attend the ritualisation of a wedding, we know what to expect and where to stand, when to be quiet and when to sing. There should be no surprises. When a priest or registrar asks the congregation if there is any cause 'or just impediment' that prevents the couple from marrying, it is very rare that there is an answer.

Ritual is performative and communicative according to Tambiah (1985).

This is not the place for an extended discussion of ritual, apart from acknowledging that ritual performances have been an inspiration for theatre practitioners throughout history – and remain so to the present day. Our multicultural society gives enormous opportunities for sharing ritual and celebrations, and dramatherapists have also developed ritual practices in their work. Schechner suggests that ritual is the focus of a convergence of anthropological, biological and aesthetic theory (Schechner, 1991). I maintain that the therapeutic experience of theatre can be compared with the performance of a healing ritual which maintains us or assists us to return to well being.

However, contemporary and 'high-tech' medicine seems to have lost its ritual roots. I was asked to work in a high tech teaching hospital with the aim of 'humanising' obstetrics. I taught theatre and anthropology to medical students and facilitated drama groups for people with fertility difficulties. The real difficulty turned out to be that as many people were getting pregnant in the drama groups as were conceiving through medical treatment. I was made to leave for 'economic reasons' – a paradox indeed!

> More needs she the divine than the physician
> (Shakespeare, *Macbeth* 5, i,70)

My Own Perspective

It must sound like a contradiction to talk about dramatic reality! How can drama be real? The media is more and more intent on creating 'reality' by recruiting 'ordinary' people for soaps, putting people in an environment away from home to create 'entertainment' or setting up chat shows for people to enact their troubled relationships before audiences. Acting for real gets the viewers. The paradox is that it is not real at all: it is contrived. It pretends to be 'real', but is actually a quick fix of emotion that stirs the viewers because it creates the illusion that these people are just like us.

The displays of emotion have to be increasingly extreme in order to surprise us: we want to react in surprise and disbelief. Domesticity has become entertainment, especially if it involves a media star or extreme violence or traumatised children or brimming emotion. Instant reaction, like fast food and ever-ready sex means that we have abolished waiting. Developmental stages are compressed into one *wow!*

Audiences become involved in these public dramas and write to characters in soaps as if they were friends or neighbours, calling them by the name of their character. Popular television drama is like an extension of our family or street; it is there in the sitting room. But nobody writes 'Dear Hamlet, I think you need to sort things out with your mother'.

We Need Surprises

I am proposing that through drama and theatre we can surprise ourselves: through *re-staging* our lives through play texts and stories, we can discover a new view of ourselves, and of the world around us. My belief is:

> Theatre art both keeps us sane and also brings us back from madness.

We talk about the different stages of our lives; I propose that we can re-stage our lives through techniques and processes of theatre art. We can address issues that are unclear or unhappy and re-stage our life is a new way. We can let go of past stages that are unhelpful and move on to a new scene or script.

By performing scenes from theatre text and through improvisation, we can get a deeper understanding and insight into our own lives. It is through metaphor and symbol that we are able to travel on creative journeys and explore new landscapes. However, it is important that the text or story or ritual creates a distance, which enables us to come closer.

It is also important for these performances to be witnessed by an audience. The performances are part of the creative process of therapeutic drama and play. My own personal journey through theatre was a journey 'from the frozen to the free'; dark times held me in dismal landscapes and I was trapped in prescribed roles at work and play. Years of therapy created new traps, then years of theatre took me on the journey to freedom. My personal stages have enabled me to understand a little more about our personal theatres, and strengthened my conviction that it is possible to 're-stage' one's life. The play can have a new and surprising ending.

Speak the speech, I pray you, as I pronounced it to you, trippingly on the tongue. But if you mouth it as many of our players do, I had as lief the town crier spoke my lines. Nor do saw the air too much with your hand, thus. But use all gently. For in the very torrent, tempest, and as I may say, whirlwind of your passion, you must acquire and beget a temperance that may give it smoothness.

(Shakespeare, *Hamlet* 3, ii, 1–8)

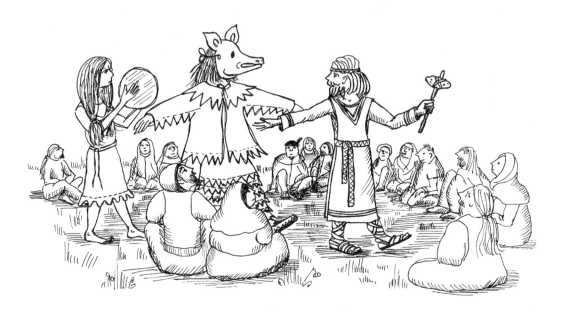

CHAPTER 2

The Play of Life and the Drama of Life

T HIS CHAPTER IS CONCERNED WITH a paradox: the reality of play and drama in living and why it is important for people 'at risk'. There is a description of different kinds of groups who could find it beneficial and some 'starter exercises' to smooth our way in if we are new to this type of work.

Play and Drama in Everyday Life

Play and drama are activities that we engage in all our lives – in one form or another. We play sports or play the fool, we play roles to fit a situation and we dress up in uniforms, we speak in an authoritative voice in one situation and then become meek and mild in another. These are just a few ways in which we create interactive activities and dramatise situations in 'non-theatrical' life. The 'Play of Life' and the 'Drama of Life' are everyday stages of human development and being. They commence even before we are born and they continue from birth until death. However this development can be disrupted by early trauma, neglect, abuse and ignorance.

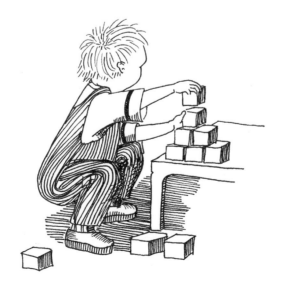

When we are playing we are repeating things that give us pleasure, we test new things and experiment, we imitate the adults around us and enact stories that we have read or seen on television. Through play we are constantly learning and acquiring new skills, testing our limits and expanding our imagination.

> Play is essential for healthy development and playfulness is the first quality
> of our early attachment with our mothers.
> (Jennings, 2005b)

Indeed we now know that the quality of the playfulness during pregnancy and early in life has a strong influence on the mental and physical health of the growing child. The pregnant woman who has time to sing and croon to her baby, rock in a rhythm and massage, tell stories and play games, is already communicating an ambience of creative playfulness to her child. It is important that this should continue during the early years.

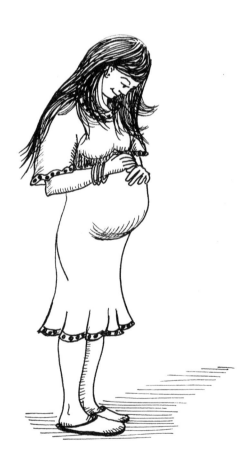

The 'playful attachment' is the significant relationship between mother and infant within which the infant is recognised: it involves father from time to time. Recognition is crucial for the child's emergent identity: to be seen in your own right and not as an appendage or extension or something (some thing) to be looked after by another. Healthy development is based on this experience of social playfulness from a very early age. Children who are deprived do not thrive, and the deprivation is not only living without enough food or fluid or warmth; it is living without social play, without the playful nurture that comes from the playful 'other' and the playful 'others'.

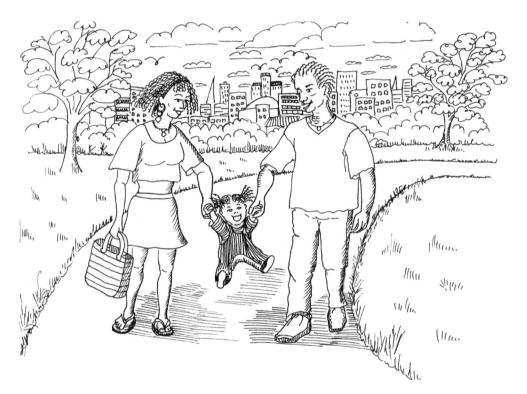

Play, Drama and Development

Play and drama are not only aspects of cultural and social development, they also have a biological basis (Schechner, 1991; Jennings, 1999; Cozolino, 2002); I would suggest that the need to dramatise is a primary drive, which is necessary for survival. I must emphasise that:

> Playfulness and dramatisation are primary drives, which are essential for survival.

We can recall children who fail to thrive because no one plays with them; there is no social interaction. Pregnant women begin dramatic scenarios in special speech with their unborn children: they talk to them and then answer themselves as if they are the infant (Jennings, 1998) – a clear example of role-reversal, or taking the role of the other. By playing the role of someone else we learn more about ourselves and we also understand more about other people: we develop empathy.

From birth, infants are constantly developing the capacity to mimic and play roles and it would seem that it is a biological imperative to have this role flexibility; we need it in order to develop resilience (Jennings, 1999). We need to be flexible towards different situations, both unknown and known. My own research has led me to propound that, parallel to all other developmental stages (such as social, physical and emotional), we also pass through dramatic development in several stages.

These broad 'staging posts' commence at birth: Embodiment–Projection–Role (EPR) (Jennings, 1990, 1998, 1999, 2004a). Children pass through these three stages of physical play (E), projective play (P) and dramatic play (R) by the time they are seven years old, and continue to engage with them in various ways through to adulthood. If we do not pass through these stages then there are difficulties with healthy attachments, maturation and the development of our imagination (Jennings, 2004d, 2005a, 2005b).

People may say that this is all very well for a western society where there is time for play! It has been suggested that an understanding of playing is a recent idea and that it fits with the increase in leisure in capitalist societies. However, I would maintain that playing in relation has always existed in all societies, and most children pass through the EPR stages. In traditional societies participation in the culture and communal ritual of the society is a part of children's development.

When I carried out my research with the Senoi Temiar people in Malaysia in 1995, I found that small children are present at the singing and dancing séances, small infants are carried on the back, infants try to assist the musicians and spend time copying the adult dances. Infants spend a lot of time playing games that are very similar to our own: for example, 'Hello Mr Tiger' instead of

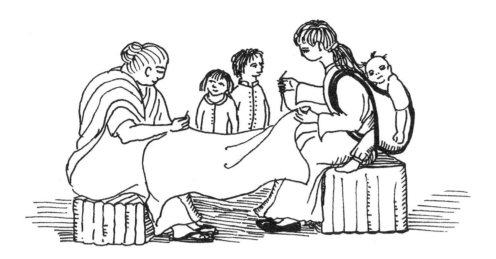

'Grandmother's Footsteps'. They also mimic adult scenes of shops, tea drinking and going into trance. Since they do not see role models of adult violence or aggression they do not display aggression in their playing (Jennings, 1995b).

Are we communicating the values of our culture and play when we take our children into busy shopping areas?

As adults it seems that we make choices of career and lifestyle based on our dominance in Embodiment or Projection or Role. These developmental

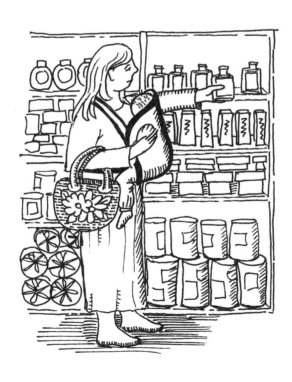

stages, I must emphasise, are our stages of dramatic development. We are born dramatised and it is the gradual understanding of 'dramatic reality' and 'everyday reality' that signals our maturity. Small children do not distinguish between 'let's pretend' and 'this is real'.

These stages take us through dramatic play to drama and theatre, from which some people will choose a theatre career – a 'role' career – and continue to create theatre on our behalf.

As adults we may need to revisit the stages of EPR: for example if we find ourselves trapped in bodies that we or others abuse, or discover that we have fixed roles that we did not choose. Play and drama based on this developmental framework forms the core of this book and its application with adults who are considered to be 'at risk'.

Will Adults Play?

Some people suggest to me that play and drama are fine for children but not for adults. Adults will think that they are being treated in a childish and unacceptable way, and they prefer to take part in adult activities. We need to find ways of talking about our activities that do not demean people, and as staff we need to be prepared to join in. Do we have difficulty with the idea of playfulness ourselves? Are we anxious about 'looking silly' or 'losing dignity'? In one of my staff training workshops, some of the staff wanted to sit and listen to the importance of play and drama instead of 'doing it'. A consultant paediatrician saved the day when we got up and said, 'Come along Matron, you and I are going to play "talking toes"'.

> Always start from where people are at: and if they want to sit and tell stories that is as good a place as anywhere.
>
> (Jennings, 1973, 2004)

Perhaps the best way is to try out the ideas and see what happens.

Starter Techniques for a Drama and Play Group

Use some of the following prompts to begin the group session.

- Who saw anything interesting on the way here today?

- Has anyone read anything or heard anything that makes interesting news this week?

- Has anyone a story to tell about anything that happened this week?

- Can anyone remember a story from childhood when they disobeyed a teacher/parent/neighbour?

- Who has a favourite story that they can remember from when they were young?

- What playground games did you play as a child?

- Describe your favourite play activity when you were young.

These are very simple 'openers' that enable people to share their experiences that are connected to play and stories. Everyone has played as a child and usually can make connections with activities or toys that they enjoyed, however simple. Even the most hardened criminal can recall a fluffy rabbit that he had as a child, and can remember how important it was (and maybe still is)!

Routledge
Taylor & Francis Group

P

Embodiment Techniques

Sitting

While group members are still sitting on chairs, try the following.

- Each person in turn says his or her name and we all try to remember them. Then throw the ball to someone and say *your* name.

- Throw the ball to someone and say *their* name.

- Throw the ball to someone and say something about them: 'You are Sue and you are wearing green socks'.

- Stretch and yawn, stretching all your body.

- Repeat and make a loud noise while you yawn.

- Stretch your fingers and make them move individually.

- Gently shrug your shoulders without straining.

- Pull funny faces to loosen up your face muscles.

- Frown upwards and downwards.

- Rub your hands together to make a whooshing noise.

- Slap your thighs to make as loud a noise as possible.

- Drum the tips of your fingers on the side of your chair.

- Do the above three actions one after the other to make the sound of a downpour of rain and it gradually slackening off.

Routledge
Taylor & Francis Group

This page may be photocopied for instructional use only. *Creative Play & Drama with Adults at Risk* © Sue Jennings 2005

Embodiment Techniques
(continued)

Standing

All of the above exercises can be done standing up, and the legs can be truly stretched too. Here are some further exercises, all of which require group members to stand.

- Wrap one hand over the other (do not 'lace' the fingers as it strains the joints); stretch upwards and then forwards, keeping your shoulders down.

- Circle each of the shoulders, one at a time and then together, outwards.

- Repeat the same exercise inwards.

- Breathe deeply from the pit of the stomach and blow out through the mouth.

- Create a breathing rhythm, in through the nose and out through the mouth. Initially, breathe to a count of two, then increase it slowly up to four.

- When people are more confident you can breathe in for four, hold the breath for four, and then breathe out for four, (again, in through the nose and out through the mouth). This exercise is especially good for people who 'panic breathe' or who have asthma.

- Stand with an even balance and beat your own chest and make an 'Ahhh' sound as loud as you can: try to get your chest to vibrate.

Routledge
Taylor & Francis Group

Embodiment Techniques
(continued)

- If you have established a culture where people can touch each other in an exercise, people can drum on one another's backs, while the person being touched makes a loud vocal noise, 'Ahhhhhh'.

- Sing together a song that everyone knows: I find that more adults remember a folk or traditional song than a recent pop song.

- Sing it again and let people take it in turns to conduct the group; they can vary the pace and the level of the sound with gestures.

- Let as many people as would like to have a turn and then suggest that the non-verbal gestures of the conductor are like miming something. What else can be communicated without using words? Try the exercise as a whole group and then in pairs.

Routledge
Taylor & Francis Group

As the group gains confidence, group members start to invent their own games and make suggestions: variations on the name game; other ways of 'shaking out'; yoga breathing exercises. Be sure to include as many people's contributions as possible.

These techniques can be played to warm up all sorts of adult groups. Let's now look at some of the different groups with whom we might want to develop our drama and play.

Who Needs Play and Drama?

The first question we need to ask in a book about play and drama with adults who are thought to be 'at risk' is, 'Who are these people?' We also need to ask why they are thought to be 'at risk'. It is important that we consider the background and early development of such people. There are various groups of people who we may include: the one thing that they may share is their vulnerability. However, there may be other links between the first four groups, as follows:

- People who may have addictions of various kinds: eating disorders, drug and alcohol abuse, addiction to violent relationships.
- People with mental ill health, which may include psychiatric or personality disorders. They may be in institutions, attending day centres or in the community.
- Individuals and families with behavioural difficulties, people prone to violence and displays of aggression, those with 'attention deficit' or 'attachment deficit'.
- Individuals in forensic settings, such as prisons, secure hospitals, community service orders; lifers, petty criminals, psychopathic criminals; those who have committed crimes during psychotic episodes.

Certain institutions value drama and theatre work more than others and they are not evenly distributed throughout the country. There are dramatherapists in some hospitals and drama workers or theatre practitioners in others. For some it is a recreational activity and in certain programmes is seen as an integral part of a treatment programme. Many centres expect people to undertake 'activities', which are meant to include drama, without preparing them with any play and drama training. This is one group of people to whom I address this book: I hope it is helpful.

There are other 'learner groups' rather than 'clinical groups' for whom these methods are invaluable. I do play and drama with people with learning difficulties and with all types of disability and impairment. It is applicable with people without sight or hearing or speech. Much of our drama and play work is non-verbal and thus becomes a 'level playing field' for people who are unable to speak for various reasons. The following adult groups can all benefit from play and drama work and most of them will enjoy being part of a theatre performance as well:

- Community groups and clubs for people with strokes and other physical impairment, often sustained as a result of accidental injury.
- Social clubs for people with learning difficulties.
- Day centres and hospitals for learning impaired adults.
- Homes and day-care centres for elderly people.
- Educational and work groups for people with all degrees of learning difficulties.
- Centres for people with multiple disabilities.
- Centres and hospitals for any of the above people who may also have mental ill health.

These activities are important for adults because they:

- Give people the chance to 'rework' the stages of dramatic development that were missed or distorted when they were children.
- Integrate people into their own heritage of art and culture.
- Encourage trust and collaboration.
- Foster independence and choice.
- Maximise people's learning potential.
- Stimulate everyone's imagination and creativity.

- Enable the strengthening of identity and building of confidence and skills.
- Help to counteract institutionalisation.
- Contribute to improvement of memory.
- Affirm people's competence.
- Allow for risk taking and exploration.
- Integrate difference at all levels.
- Allow people to experience the effects of their actions.
- Allow people to play with ideas and outcomes.
- Reinstate the importance of the arts both for society as well as for the individual.

With so many ways of looking at the phenomena of play and drama, I am sure that you can see many within your own experience. Any one of the above ideas is sufficient as an aim for the drama and play that you will develop with your groups. And don't forget, you can discuss the aims of the activities with your groups when you establish your working contract with them. The contract is the final topic to be discussed in this chapter.

A Working Contract for Drama and Play Work

Generally speaking I think that contracts should be in writing for each person or at least for the group as a whole. There may be some basic elements that are in every contract and others that you and your group decide should also be included. The essential elements for the contract are also listed on Worksheet 2.1, which you can photocopy and hand out to group members.

Essential elements for your contract:

- Everyone agrees to be punctual and to stay to the end of the session.
- Everyone makes a commitment to attend the agreed number of sessions.

- In the case of essential absence, such as illness, the drama worker needs to be notified as early as possible.
- Physical and verbal violence is not permitted in the group – unless it is necessary within a dramatic role.
- Bullying, racism and any other forms of discrimination are not permitted.
- Group members agree to listen to each other and not 'over-talk'.
- Group members agree to show each other respect, affirmation, tolerance and support.
- If group members share personal material about their lives, it remains confidential within the group.

Members may want to modify, clarify or use other words for the contract and to add other conditions. Sanctions may be suggested by group members for people who break the rules.

Establishing the contract is a social skills activity in itself. It can form the first session and may encourage debate and discussion. It is important that everyone's suggestion is heard. Contracts can be reviewed and modified at any time with the agreement of the group. With some groups it may be necessary to restate the terms each week so they become internalised and reinforced.

Everything can be explored through the drama and actionwork, even the contract:

- Set up a 'debating society' exercise to discuss the contract – with some people for the contract and some against.
- Imagine you are in a court and the items have to be teased out before being agreed.
- Write each item of the contract on a small piece of paper: everyone pulls one out of the hat and describes why it is important.
- Set the contract to music: for example, to the tune of 'New York, New York…' ('Contract, Contract…'!). It may sound silly, but if people want to play they may well be inspired! And it is a very good way of learning, too!

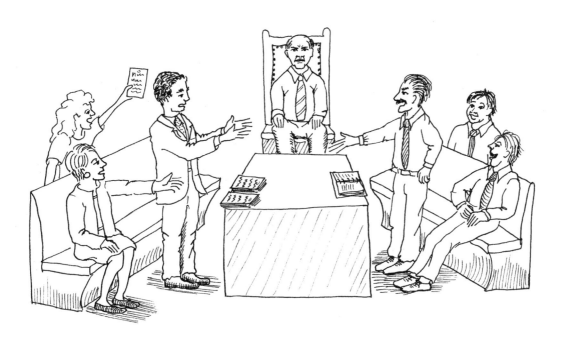

They could be debating the contract on a grand scale!

Worksheet 2.1
Contract for the Drama Group

Name _____ Date _____

Essential elements for your contract:

- Everyone agrees to be punctual and to stay to the end of the session.
- Everyone makes a commitment to attend the agreed number of sessions.
- In the case of essential absence, such as illness, the drama worker needs to be notified as early as possible.
- Physical and verbal violence is not permitted in the group – unless it is necessary within a dramatic role.
- Bullying, racism and any other forms of discrimination are not permitted.
- Group members agree to listen to each other and not 'over-talk'.
- Group members agree to show each other respect, affirmation, tolerance and support.
- If group members share personal material about their lives, it remains confidential within the group.

Read through the contract carefully and add below any further items that you think are important.

_____

_____

_____

_____

Signature of participant _____ **Date** _____
Signature of drama worker _____

Worksheet 2.2
Your Life in Play and Drama

Name _____ Date _____

> Close your eyes and think about play and drama in
> your own life, especially when you were a child.
> Then answer the following questions as a way of
> reminding yourself about your own playful life.

1 Did you ever do drama in your teens? If so, was it fun
   or scary?

   _____

2 What were your favourite games in your teens?

   _____

3 What were your favourite stories in your teens?

   _____

4 Can you remember games and drama when you were
   younger?

   _____

5 What did you play at when you were small?

   _____

6 Did you have favourite stories when you were a small
   child?

   _____

> Think about these experiences and try to recall some
> good memories.
> Share anything from your past playfulness with the group,
> and see whether you have neglected to play as an adult.

You can continue your answers on the back of this sheet.

CHAPTER 3

Ancient Wisdom for Changing Times

I N MY OWN WORK OF 're-staging', which is a form of theatre-for-change, as well as in dramatherapy, I often use Shakespeare as a starting point for an understanding of madness, dreams, politics, violence, conflict, love, nightmares and daydreams.

Shakespeare deals with envy, jealousy, grief, ambivalence, horror, fear, fury, sex, in profound ways that connect with all of us as human beings. I also use other texts, especially from the Ancient Greeks, and I turn many myths and legends into dramatic form. Through participation in a workshop or performance, people not only *feel* differently; they also *think* differently. Issues that seem insurmountable, landscapes that appear bleak and conflicts that threaten to destroy all take on new dimensions through a theatre experience.

First Principles of Drama and Theatre

Let us return to some first principles of drama and theatre. Theatre is a paradox: it is something 'out there', unconnected to our day-to-day lives; we say that it is distanced from us; yet through witnessing or participating in theatre, we can come closer to our hopes, fears and dilemmas.

It is indeed a paradox to say that 'something distanced enables greater closeness'. The Greeks knew that theatre was crucial to the well-being of society and would contribute to stability. The word 'theatre', or *theatron*, has the same root as *theoria* (theory): therefore there was the idea that we go to the theatre to understand things. *Theatron* also has the same root as *theos* (god): thus in the theatre we can be in touch with the divine and the sublime. Theatre and its associated roots have multiple meanings, which integrate theatre as a central influence with society.

The theatre of Ancient Greece, as well as Shakespeare's plays, provide us with many stories and ideas, too. They also allow us to extend ourselves because we have to communicate to a lot of people. Modern living is often very cramped and confined, and many of today's theatres are small. By contrast, the stadium or amphitheatre was usually where most Ancient Greek dramas were enacted, and often they could get out of control. Imagining that we are moving and speaking in a vast space can help us to 'expand', at least through our imaginations.

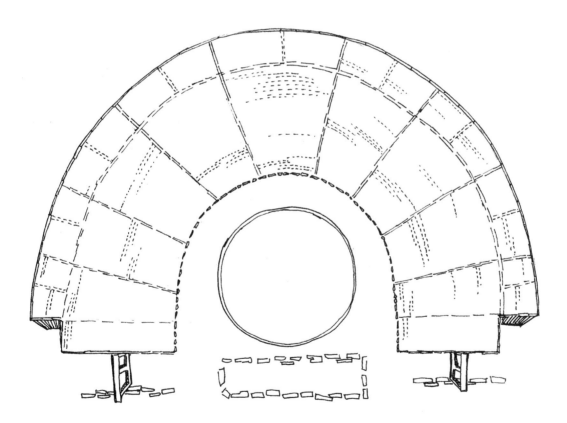

Theatre is the most integrative of the art forms because it includes dance, ritual, mime, puppetry, masks, set and light design, music and text (Jennings, 1986, 1990). This integration allows as much flexibility as possible for participants, with variations in artistic techniques and methods.

We must not neglect the aesthetic of theatre, which perhaps is difficult to find in instant entertainment. The coming together of the many parts into an artistic whole gives us an aesthetic experience: we say that it 'works', that it is 'truthful' or 'authentic', that it 'communicates' to us. The healing metaphors enable us to experience transformation in our inner lives as well as with the group as a whole. Indeed the embedding in our physical bodies of important symbols and metaphors allows this transformation to take place. These symbols are there at our disposal and become a reservoir of health, which we can call upon when we feel unwell. The physical core of our experience is the dominant medium for the resting place of the symbols.

The Paradox of Hamlet

This artistic truth is paradoxical because it is a fiction enacted by a group of performers. Hillman (1983) suggests that poetry and stories are healing fictions, that are necessary for transformation – and that they are healing *because* they are fictions. Paradoxically, Hamlet castigates himself because the actor can express his emotions freely, yet he cannot.

> Is it not monstrous that this player here,
> But in a fiction, in a dream of passion,
> Could force his soul so to his own conceit
> That, from her working, all his visage wann'd;
> Tears in his eyes, distraction in's aspect,
> A broken voice....
> (Shakespeare, *Hamlet* 3, i, 558–563)

This is a very interesting discussion to have with the group because through our drama work we believe that people can access their feelings and find ways to express them; it is possible to work 'from the outside in', and the safe structure of a play or story allows us to do that. It is after this speech of Hamlet's that he decides to put on a play in order to 'catch the conscience' of his uncle, whom he believes has murdered his older brother (Hamlet's father).

> The play's the thing
> Wherein I'll catch the conscience of the king
> (Shakespeare, *Hamlet* 2, ii, 14–15)

Shakespeare and Madness

Several Shakespearean plays explore the theme of madness in its many forms. Among them are *Hamlet, King Lear, Richard III, Macbeth* and *The Winter's Tale*. Hamlet says that he is going to feign madness in order to gain evidence that his uncle murdered his father, but by the middle of the play we are left with a question of *who* is really mad? Towards the end of the play, Ophelia has a complete nervous breakdown and speaks as if she is psychotic.

King Lear slowly deteriorates and his family are unable to cope with him. Richard III is in modern terminology a psychopathic killer, whose ambition to be king drives him to murder anyone that stands in his way. Macbeth, driven by his wife, has similar ambitions: like Richard III, he employs contract killers.

The Winter's Tale

In *The Winter's Tale*, we see the mental breakdown of Leontes the king; Paulina is trying to calm him and allow him to sleep; she suggests that his other visitors, who creep around him and sigh, actually keep him awake!

> I come to bring him sleep. 'Tis such as you,
> That creep like shadows by him, and do sigh
> At each his needless heavings – such as you
> Nourish the cause of his awakening. I
> Do come with words as medicinal as true,
> Honest, as either, to purge him of that humour
> That presses him from sleep.
> (Shakespeare, *The Winter's Tale* 2, iii, 33–41)

The Winter's Tale is a journey through madness and jealousy, forbearance and forgiveness. The 'winter' in the title is the winter of King Leontes' madness, his tortuous journey through his jealousy and the destruction of his family. His young son eventually pines away, whereas at the beginning of the play he was playful and a storyteller. His father says to him:

> Go play, boy, play: thy mother plays, and I
> Play too –
> (Shakespeare, *The Winter's Tale* 1, ii, 187–8)

As You Like It

Shakespeare is a genius at presenting the layers of meaning in the word 'play', of writing about the 'play within the play', of finding metaphors for life through the metaphor of the actor. Perhaps this speech by Jacques in *As You Like It* is the one we know best.

> All the world's a stage,
> And all the men and women merely players;
> They have their exits and their entrances,
> And one man in his time plays many parts,
> (Shakespeare, *As You Like It* 2, vii,140–143)

What do we think about this statement? Maybe we can explore it with the group in discussion. (Use Worksheet 3.1). Maybe the first line can be the title of our group!

Take the whole speech that describes the stages of life from Jacques' point of view, read through the stages and invite comments. Each person can say the lines to describe a stage. You can use the stages to sculpt or improvise (see below), and see whether people would change them for their own description.

Do we agree with Shakespeare's constant use of theatre and the actor to describe our lives and living?

The Importance of Comedy

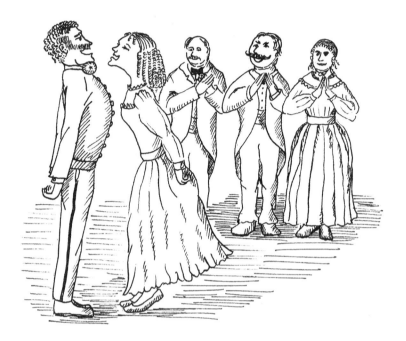

The following story can be easily divided for use in a variety of workshops and can act as a blueprint for other stories and their exploration. Allow as much discussion as possible around ideas and themes, and start with small manageable pieces.

There is an old tale, first told by Ovid, that is a lot of fun: the story of King Midas. It has several versions and can form the basis of several drama workshops. The following is the full story, followed by a range of exercises that will help you to explore the content in many ways. These exercises can then be adapted for other material.

The Story of King Midas

In ancient times, Apollo, the god of music and medicine, challenges the trickster god, Pan to a musical competition. They invite King Midas to be the judge, and there is a group of rather silly giggling nymphs who are watching the proceedings.

Pan's music is rough and rugged, rhythmic and rousing; it reminds everyone of his earthy approach to life and love. Pan lives at the margins of the forest and is known as the goat god because of his cloven hooves; he seduces women with his Pan pipes. The competition starts and he plays his music first as the nymphs swoon and giggle together.

Apollo also has an instrument – his lyre – and he gently draws his fingers across the strings. His music is sweet, coming from the deepest source: the soul. Apollo can leave his lyre hanging from a tree and the breeze plays sweet music as it blows through the strings. However, the nymphs take little notice of Apollo's music.

When both the musicians have finished everyone looks expectantly at King Midas. They are aghast when he awards the prize to Pan. Pan is smiling and bowing, not realising that Apollo is incandescent with rage. Midas turns to him in horror, and freezes on the spot as Apollo points his hand at him and presses it down – the sign of giving a curse. He does not say a word and Midas hurries off, desperate to get away.

On his way home, Midas keeps scratching his head, and shaking it from side to side. He is exhausted when he arrives at his palace and goes straight to his room. He looks in his mirror and looks over his shoulder to see if there is someone else in the room – he does not recognise his own reflection! He has grown an enormous and grisly pair of ass's ears. He cannot believe what he sees: the punishment of Apollo.

He immediately gets a turban and swathes it round and round his ears so that no one can see them. He summons the palace barber and tells him that he is the only person allowed to see his 'growth' and he swears him to secrecy. Once a month the barber comes to the palace, removes the turban and trims the hair on King Midas's ears as well as the rest of his hair and beard. The barber finds the whole thing rather amusing, and smiles to himself as he snips.

However, after a few months he finds that the burden of keeping the secret is becoming very heavy. When he goes home to his wife and she asks him about his day, the barber is about to tell her – and then stops short. She presses him and then becomes suspicious when he changes the subject! He is bursting to tell someone and it is getting worse!

The next time he goes to the palace, after he has cut and trimmed he goes out of the back door, looks on either side of him and makes for the river. He kneels down on the bank and scrapes up a piece of earth, and he whispers, 'Ass's ears, ass's ears, King Midas has ass's ears, King Midas has ass's ears!' He replaces the earth and pats it down and goes home, very relieved.

And the rushes of the river blow gently in the breeze and rustle in their leaves, 'King Midas has ass's ears, Midas has ass's ears'. And the stream trills over the stones and sings, 'King Midas has ass's ears, ass's ears…'

And so a private secret is carried to the whole world along the streams and rivers and everyone knows about King Midas and the revenge of Apollo.

Exploration of Stories Using Drama Games

Once you have read or told the story to the group, you can play some drama games to warm up and to get to know the story. The games can be used to warm up the group in different sessions, and you can slowly add your own exercises and encourage group members to bring their own.

Basically you are using these techniques to:

- Physically 'warm up' the group, ready for action (see also Hickson, 1995).
- Encourage people to collaborate as a group.
- Stimulate the imagination in a fun way.

- Sow the seeds of creativity.
- Gradually build confidence.
- Develop trust within the group.
- Expand people's potential beyond their usual limits.
- Create structures within which people feel safe to improvise.
- Allow for contributions and group innovation.

Drama Games

- Everyone has a good 'shake out', a stretch and a yawn. Walk briskly around the room taking care not to bump into anyone; speed the walk up and slow it down.
- Everyone touches the four corners of the room, claps their hands twice and touches three pairs of knees, as fast as possible. Then tell everyone to retrace their steps, remembering all the knees they touched!
- Stand in a circle, hold hands and 'invisibly' pass a squeeze round the circle. Then pass a squeeze in the other direction and see if they can cross over without being seen!
- Put on a CD of a jazz band and everyone mimes playing an instrument or conducting; do the same with a piece of classical music.
- Everyone imagines they are playing an enormous musical instrument, then a tiny instrument that they can barely hold. Choose different types of music: brass band, pop, dance music, and so on.
- Practise humming until your lips tingle; share a song that everyone can sing together.

Developing Themes from a Story
Using the EPR Framework

If you explore small chunks of a story (or play or poem) in various ways, it enables people to:

- Take in a piece of the story at a time without being overwhelmed.
- Go deeper into a character or an interaction, at a gradual pace.
- Remove the anxiety about 'performing' or having to remember words or produce a 'product'.

- Integrate different aspects of themselves: physically, as well as emotionally and reflectively.
- Pursue different ideas: there is no single answer that is 'right'!
- Allow people to discover their own ideas and interpretations of what a scene or character or is about.

The following are some ways for exploring the Midas story – you can adapt them to any text that you want, although care needs to be taken in the choice of stories: there are guidelines for this choice laid down in most dramatherapy books. I use an EPR framework to plan the session. Therefore it will include some physical exploration in addition to the warm-up (E); some projective ideas such as painting or drawing (P); some role techniques through improvisation (R). This creates a developmental structure for each individual as well as the group as a whole. It is very important to provide opportunities to develop the voice.

> It is important to remember that you need to know the story very well indeed and that you have checked it out for possible sensitive or dangerous themes.
> (Jennings, 2004d)

> I always make a point of using a story where there is a theme of transformation and some kind of resolution at the end.
> (Jennings, 2004d)

Embodiment
- Musical Characters (with or without music): group members walk around the room until you call, 'Freeze!' as a signal to stop. You then say the name of a character and everyone creates it (otherwise known as a 'sculpt'). For example, you can call out: giggling nymphs; Pan and his rough music; whispering rushes; the barber bursting with the secret. Keep the pace brisk! (E). Afterwards, people walk around the room again, as before.

- Mime the scene where Midas slowly becomes aware that he is growing huge ears – once it dawns on him, he then covers them up in shame (E).
- Sculpt different characters in pairs as they interact with one another (E).
- Choose a character from the story and explore how he or she walks, sits, or greets others. Imagine the costume that the character might be wearing, how does it affect his or her posture and gestures? (E).
- What voice does this character have? Play with different sounds before using words (E).
- Have a conversation with another character just using sounds (E).

Projection
- Paint a picture of the landscape of the river and the rushes (P).
- Draw or paint a picture of King Midas with his ears! (P).

Role
- In pairs, create the scene between the barber and King Midas: the barber is trying not to laugh (R).
- In pairs, create the scene between the barber and his wife, as she tries to wheedle the secret out of him (R).
- In small groups, create the scene of the competition and the curse (R).
- Think of other contexts for the story – for example, what would happen in a modern setting? Improvise the different ideas in small groups (R).
- Tell and enact the story from the point of view of the nymphs or a servant at the palace (R). If this is a writing exercise it is (P).
- Enact the whole story without words (R).
- Improvise your own words for the story (R).
- Enact the whole story with words – and include the sound effects of the musicians, the rushes and the river (R).

Leave time for discussion of the story. Talk about how people feel about the different characters: for whom do they have most sympathy?

A Midsummer Night's Dream

The story of King Midas contains the same story that Shakespeare used for one of the themes (transformation with an ass's head) in *A Midsummer Nights Dream* (Act III). You may think of taking the same scene from that play and exploring it and then comparing it with Midas.

The scene occurs when the workmen are rehearsing their play to perform at the palace for Theseus' wedding celebrations. The king of the fairies, Oberon, wants to exact revenge on the queen, Titania, by making her fall in love with something monstrous. Puck, his henchman, puts an ass's head on one of the actors (whose name is Bottom), and Oberon puts a love potion on Titania's eyes so she falls in love with Bottom when she wakes. You can explore this scene in groups of four (Oberon, Titania, Puck and Bottom) or go to the original text and implore the rhythmic language. If you improvise the scene first, the text will seem less scary.

Act 3 opens with the workmen rehearsing their play; Puck comes in to watch and then puts the ass's head on Bottom as he is waiting to make his entrance. All the workmen flee as he approaches and he is very puzzled. Titania then wakes, sees him, and addresses him as a lover, which puzzles him even more! It is a fun scene to enact and can be explored with a variety of masks, or just a mask for the ass's head.

The play as a whole is therapeutic. Although it starts with family and marital conflict between various couples, the key players run away to the forest, there are various tricks (and, at times, gratuitous violence) in the woods – there are resolutions at the end. The workmen and their play-within-a-play is a key theme that is woven throughout. I have used the story and the text in forensic settings and the staff reaction initially was interesting. They said to me, 'Sue, you can't use Shakespeare – especially a story about fairies. The chaps wouldn't join in! Why not use something they all know – like Colditz (!)' However, I saturated the staff and group with the story (videos, cartoons,

Lamb's Tales from Shakespeare) and everyone without exception gained a tremendous amount from exploring the play over a period of nine months (Jennings, 1997).

While I was working in Delhi running a training course for people working with children with special needs, we took the play as an example of what could be possible. Again, people thought Shakespeare would be impossible for people with limited language and learning difficulties to understand. What was achieved was extraordinary and we put an abbreviated 'production' together in two weeks that we showed at the British Council. Showing the play was important politically, because no-one had thought it possible! However, we have to be very careful about public performances with vulnerable people.

Performance

Performance is the culmination of all drama, it is the point at which drama becomes theatre. I believe in this sharing of our work. However, the product should not take over from the process when we are using drama with people with special needs. It may be that we perform our work to each other, to a group of staff or to another ward. It may be that we can perform within the context of a festival at the hospital or school, or maybe there can be a Christmas pantomime or a Diwali ritual.

However, it is really important that we feel we can work with drama and theatre *without* the pressure on ourselves or the group that it has to culminate in a performance. Some role-plays and improvisations have aims in their own right; we will have sessions when we want to play with ideas as part of the development of themes.

If we are working specifically towards a performance (as contrasted perhaps with the idea of a sharing or presentation), then we can involve more creative processes and other people as well. This will be addressed throughout Chapter 10, but as Titania says towards the end of the play:

First rehearse your song by rote,
To each word a warbling note.
Hand in hand with fairy grace
Will we sing and bless this place.
(Shakespeare, *A Midsummer Nights Dream* 5, i, 360–390)

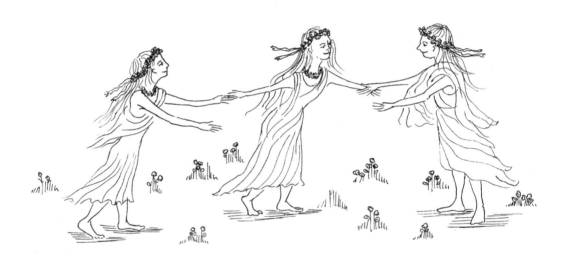

Worksheet 3.1
All the World's a Stage

Name _____ Date _____

> All the world's a stage
> And all the men and women merely players.
> They have their exits and their entrances,
> And one man in his time plays many parts,
> His acts being seven ages. At first the infant,
> Mewling and puking in the nurse's arms.
> Then the whining schoolboy with his satchel
> Ands shining morning face, creeping like snail
> Unwillingly to school. And then the lover,
> Sighing like a furnace, with a woeful ballad
> Made to his mistress' eyebrow. Then, a soldier,
> Full of strange oaths, and bearded like the pard,
> Jealous in honour, sudden, and quick in quarrel,
> Seeking the bubble reputation
> Even in the cannon's mouth. And then the justice,
> In fair round belly with good capon lined,
> With eyes severe and beard of formal cut,
> Full of wise saws and modern instances;
> And so he plays his part. The sixth age shifts
> Into the lean and slippered pantaloon,
> With spectacles on nose and pouch on side,
> His youthful hose, well saved, a world too wide
> For his shrunk shank, and his big, manly voice,
> Turning again toward childish treble, pipes
> And whistles in his sound. Last scene of all,
> That ends this strange eventful history,
> Is second childishness and mere oblivion,
> Sans teeth, sans eyes, sans taste, sans everything.
>
> (Shakespeare, *As You Like It* 2, vii, 140–143)

Read through this whole speech, which is about the different stages in a person's life.
Think about each stage and whether or not you would change it to fit your own experience.

_____

_____

You can continue your answer on the back of this sheet.

Routledge Taylor & Francis Group

Worksheet 3.2
Random Poems A

Name _____ Date _____

WHOW!

Golden threads excite stars!

Where am I going asks ......?

Trackers?

Smith for Leader!

Bump in the night scares birds!

Love is all you need.

The colour is green

Is that what we want?

Hello again Mr Alien!

Hidden Landscape

My favourite fish

Write any of the phrases above to make a nonsense poem
and decorate it with colours.

_____

_____

_____

_____

Read your poem to the group as if it is serious.

You can continue your poem on the back of this sheet.

Worksheet 3.3
Random Poems B

Name _____ Date _____

Look through a range of newspapers and magazines.
Cut out phrases and headlines to create your own poem,
including the title.
Use the space below to plan your poem.
Decorate the final version to make a scroll.
You can read your poem to the group or ask someone
else to read it.

CHAPTER 4

Games, Games and Yet More Games

THE ONE THING THAT ALL types of games have in common is that they have a set of rules, and woe betide the person who breaks the rules! There are established games for teams of people and pairs, there are physical games and there are 'brain games' such as chess and dominoes. The phrase 'mind games' has particularly negative associations as is often illustrated in psychological thrillers.

The expression 'playing games' has many meanings, some of which are positive and some less so. 'You are playing games with me,' is used to describe an attempt to wrong foot someone. Maybe we want to cheat them, or maybe we seek power as a power game. These games have their own sets of rules that serve to mystify and confuse.

We are also told that it does not matter who wins a game, it is how we play it that counts: we must 'play fair' and not cheat. 'It's only a game', they say.

Countless children are damaged by game playing – for example, there are:

- Abusive games played by paedophiles ('I'm coming to get you').
- Games that cause us to be bullied because we can't second guess the rules.
- Sadistic games played by cruel parents.
- Initiation games inflicted on children by older children.
- Games that are designed to embarrass and denigrate, especially in public.
- And there is sarcasm and ridicule from sports coaches because we are not good enough at games.

However, there are lots of games that are exhilarating. They can contribute to positive growth and increase confidence. They can improve coordination and balance, flexibility and fitness.

Whatever method we use to apply games, with children or with adults, we need to be very sensitive to a person's games' experience. Our messages need to be clear: people need reassurance that they will not be made to look foolish and ground rules should be explained. It is easy to assume incorrectly that 'everyone knows this game'.

Games with a Set Format

Games form a core of the play experience – indeed it is necessary to put the two words 'play' and 'games' together. If we talk about gaming without play, we conjure up rather different activities! Children will say, 'Let's play a game about monsters,' which means they will dramatise a story that usually has a set format, as the following example illustrates.

Grandma Giant

Two of my grandchildren had a set game that they wanted to play over and over again. I had to be a monstrous giant asleep, making a lot of noise snoring. In my hand was a treasure map. They were two brave characters who wanted to take the map from the giant and find the treasure. They would slowly creep up on me and I would turn in my sleep and make more noises. Perhaps I was waking up? And they would freeze until I went still again.

I could hear the younger child, who was three years old, saying, 'Take it, you take it' to his older brother, who was four years old. The older boy was the brave character, and his younger brother wasn't too sure if it was 'just playing' or really scary. After a few attempts they managed to steal the map and then went off to find the treasure. However, the end of the scene did not matter; it was the game of trying to outwit the giant that was important.

Drama Games

Drama games are very specific warm-up games for drama and theatre work. The well-known British theatre director Clive Barker, whose recent death is a great loss to all of us in the 'games' business, wrote a superb book called *Theatre Games* (Barker, 1977). This book has a wide range of activities of all kinds and is many a group worker's essential handbook!

Dramatic Games

I am applying the word 'dramatic games' as a contrast to 'drama games' to illustrate certain types of game that seem to have their own sets of rules but are not games in the usual sense of the word. Dramatic games that are like dramatic play can be repeated more-or-less the same, over and over again and involve stock characters: mummies and daddies, cowboys and Indians, doctors and nurses, monsters and heroes, aliens and earthlings. It is like a ritualisation of a piece of drama that is a known piece. It is exactly the same for adults who have adaptations of similar set pieces that are based on familiar material. They may be scenes from 'soaps' or television game shows. Karaoke may be used as an ice-breaker as may scenes from epic films such as the battle with the Titans in *Jason and the Argonauts*. The whole story does not seem necessary for this activity; it is a particular sequence that is important. A shared moment of an event from life, sport or entertainment means that we can start with something that is familiar.

I am indebted to Andy Hickson for extensive discussions on the use of games in drama, especially in relation to re-learning programmes. Everyone has their favourite games, group leaders as well as participants, and we need to be sensitive as to whether the games are competitive or collaborative. My personal view is that we safely use both and keep the balance between the individual and the group. Whatever game is being played in the drama group, it is important that it is 'not for real'. Once it stops being 'not for real' then it ceases to be the drama group and turns into everyday life.

Set Games

When I first started drama teaching at a school of occupational therapy, the principal asked me if I would teach the students how to run a bingo session as part of their activities. I was most insulted! What had this to do with the creative work that I was developing? Why on earth should I be asked to teach games as part of drama! I was much younger then, and rather too proud of myself; how right this elderly woman was. I had a lot to learn as I went out and about, working in long-stay institutions both in the UK and overseas.

The more experienced I became, the more I began to understand that the 'set games' are such an important part of social life: whether cards, chess, dominoes or mah-jong. Hospital wards had teams and clubs, people's expertise was discussed and bets were placed. Having revisited this part of my work in long-stay psychiatric hospitals in Romania, I can again see how important these social games are in building communities and encouraging communication and relationships. Usually the people in these hospitals are sitting and rocking, pacing or staying in their rooms. There is a pervading atmosphere of institutionalisation. There is not enough funding for fresh fruit, let alone recreational resources. The first equipment that the people asked for turned out to be new packs of cards and six chess sets!

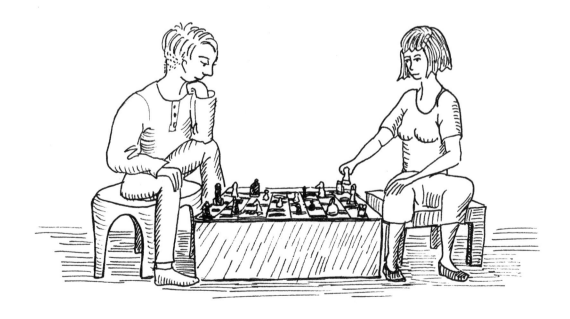

A Personal Admission

My own antipathy towards set games is something that I have avoided exploring for a very long time. It is only with the relatively recent advent of grandchildren that I have had to re-examine my avoidance of these activities. When I visit them they will often ask me to join in a card or board games, and I will always respond, why don't we do drama? So we have created plays and scenes and improvised epics together, including Shakespeare.

However I have always sensed that there is a disappointment from the children that I do not join in their games. I had to ask myself why. I have to face up to the fact that these are activities that I am not very good at: I used to joke that the only card game that I could play was Snap! But there is an enormous learning opportunity for me here as I allow myself to unravel my avoidance of set games. I am not very good at them – indeed I am hopeless! Where does that come from?

As children my siblings and I were always encouraged to be individuals and develop our own ideas – to be creative and adventurous and to break the rules if necessary. This would include the rules of conventional thinking in education, for example. The rules of 'good manners' were essential rules. This meant that some of the siblings had little schooling and where possible we did not play games. My father, by and large, did not believe in team games and would talk about 'herd instinct'. My headteacher was written to and told that I would not play hockey because it would damage my career as a dancer! There then ensued a two-year spate of letters – very polite ones. Meanwhile I had to walk round the playing field while my classmates played hockey: I was bullied and ridiculed, but that is another story.

Games of sport, I realised, are not approved of! Not only that: as a younger child I suffered agonies when we were expected to join in 'a bit of fun' at the church fete and do the three-legged race or the relay race. I became sick, I had stomach thumps and my temperature shot up.

Activities that were not encouraged became activities over which I felt conflict and therefore became ill. In turn, these became activities that I could not do – and they eventually became activities that I disapproved of!

No wonder I had no skills at sports and sporty games. It has taken me many years to understand this important childhood parental influence. So why not include bingo? It is an important dramatic ritual, as I discovered when I visited the weekly bingo session where I live now. Groups of people meet, catch up on the news and at the same time they have some fun and maybe win a prize. You do not go there as a lone player!

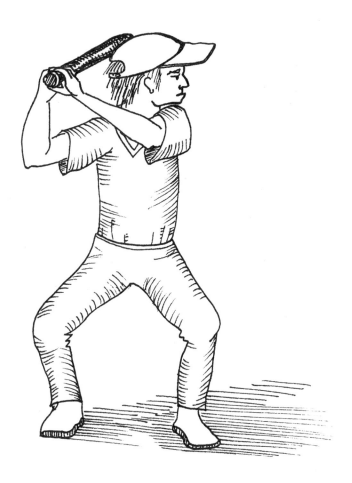

Summary of Different Types of Games

Drama games: various movement and voice games to help 'warm-up' the group ready for creative work. They expand everyone's potential.

Dramatic games: repeated games from childhood, with stock characters, slices of life and television, very good starters before getting into drama work.

Set games: a range of activities that can include: all types of sports, board and card games, team and pair games, party games and playground games.

Activities

The following pages contain a wide selection of games – some competitive, some collaborative – all to be played with a sense of fun.

Balloon and Ball Games

- Each group member blows up a balloon and then everyone tries to keep the balloons in the air at the same time.

- Try to keep a beach ball in the air with the whole group.

- Two teams pat a beach ball or a large balloon over a net, keeping it in the air.

- Bounce a beach ball so it is high enough for the person bouncing it to have time to run across the circle before it comes down again.

- Make a tunnel of legs and roll a ball from one end to the other.

- Pass a balloon between one another using only your knees.

- Pass an orange between one another using only your knees.

- Balance a balloon on the palm of your hand and give it to a partner.

- Place a balloon between you and your partner and try and burst it.

- Walk with beach balls on your head.

- Bounce a 'high bounce' ball and someone else has to catch it.

Routledge Taylor & Francis Group

P This page may be photocopied for instructional use only. *Creative Play & Drama with Adults at Risk* © Sue Jennings 2005

Balloon and Ball Games
(continued)

Imaginary Balloon or Ball Games

- Blow up an imaginary balloon and hand it to someone else.

- Blow up an imaginary balloon, tie a string to it and fly it like a kite.

- Juggle with imaginary balls; then do the same with a partner.

- Bounce a ball in a circle and develop as many variations as possible – other people can guess which ball game you are playing.

- Imagine you have a piece of clay in your hand and slowly you are modelling a very small ball the size of a table tennis ball. Then it grows bigger like a tennis ball, then even larger like a football. Smooth it very carefully. Finally 'dribble' the ball around the room, making sure you do not bump into anyone else.

- Imagine you have a football and practise your footballing skills with a partner.

- In slow motion, have an imaginary five-a-side football game, always watching where the 'ball' is: this is very good for concentration! If the group is bigger you can involve 'the crowd', again in slow motion, as they respond to the match.

- In small groups, improvise any games of sports without using language: use only non-verbal communication.

Balloon and Ball Games
(continued)

- Have a sports festival with every group creating a different sport: you have only imaginary equipment. If it is a large group, you can create the non-verbal Olympics.

- If the group can work verbally without getting out of control, then add words – for the sports festival and for the Olympics.

Routledge
Taylor & Francis Group

Newspaper Games

Newspapers are the cheapest form of equipment that you can possibly obtain – and all the paper can be recycled afterwards. When the games refer to the contents of the newspapers, make sure you have a wide variety of magazines as well as papers.

In addition you will need several pairs of scissors, rolls of masking tape and a decorative bowl or box for 'lucky dip' exercises. Rhythmic music or a drum are needed for the games that are similar to 'musical chairs'.

- Everyone stands on a single piece of newspaper. Then, to music or a drum beat, everyone walks around the room until the sound stops, when they must stand on the nearest piece of newspaper. You take one piece away – they start walking again. People drop out as the number of sheets is reduced, until only one is left. The advantage of using newspapers is that people have to exercise a lot of care so that they do not get ripped!

- Divide into groups of three or four people. Put one sheet of paper on the floor for each group. Use the drum beat or music again, but after each round the newspaper is torn in half. The group members have to be inventive in terms of how they can stand on the paper when the sound stops!

Routledge
Taylor & Francis Group

P

Newspaper Games
(continued)

- Cut out some long headlines and then cut them into individual words. Put them in a box and invite everyone to take one word. Find who else belongs to your headline. Make the whole phrase on the floor and see if everyone has made the original headlines.

- Cut out some words from newspapers and magazines and mix them in the box. Each small group takes a handful: can you make a sentence that uses all the words?

- Create a crazy advertisement from different newspaper words.

- Scrumple up small pieces of newspaper and use them to fight a fun battle.

- Scrumple up large pieces of newspaper; use masking tape to keep them in place and use them as a football.

- Make a newspaper mask by tearing two eye-holes in a sheet. Play a game of monsters and mayhem: you are not allowed to hold your mask in place and your partner has to try and blow your mask off.

- Lie under a 'blanket' of newspapers – and try to get out without making any sound.

- Tear out words from the newspaper and then mime them for others to guess.

Routledge Taylor & Francis Group

P This page may be photocopied for instructional use only. *Creative Play & Drama with Adults at Risk* © Sue Jennings 2005

Status Games

This term originated with Keith Johnstone and he describes these games in his excellent book *Impro: Improvisation and the Theatre* (Johnstone, 1981). He points out how often we use status games in our conversations and interactions. For example, he describes the following:

A: What are you reading?

B: *War and Peace.*

A: Ah! That's my favourite book!

The person A had been told to respond in a low status way to the answer and we can see how it answered in a high status. So if they did it again they could have given a low status response:

A: What are you reading?

B: *War and Peace.*

A: Ah! That's my favourite book!

B: Really?

A: Oh yes. Of course, I only look at the pictures.

The group can get intense enjoyment from exploring the ideas of status games and then creating their own (see Worksheets 4.1 and 4.2). The games can involve conversations between any two people who seem to have the same status and each one tries to get the edge on the other. You may need to make some ground rules to start with by stating, 'Person A is keeping in high status and Person B in low status'. Then bring in variations, so that they can shift position.

It is also interesting to look at unequal partners such as the prince and the beggar, and let them respond in reverse expectation. (See and use Worksheet 4.1.) Johnstone gives us this example:

> Tramp: 'Ere, where are you going?
> Duchess: I'm sorry, I didn't quite catch …
> Tramp: Are you deaf as well as blind?

He makes the point that status is something that one *does*, not something that one necessarily *is*. He suggests that people become friends when they can agree to play status games together. For example, if I can say to a friend, 'Well you old bag, where are you off to?', there is an explicit agreement that we can play status games together. She does not say to me, 'Watch who you are calling a bag!'

Encourage the people in your groups to observe and recognise status games. Use Worksheets 4.1 and 4.2 with the group. Status games are played between politicians, between television interviewers and interviewees, between

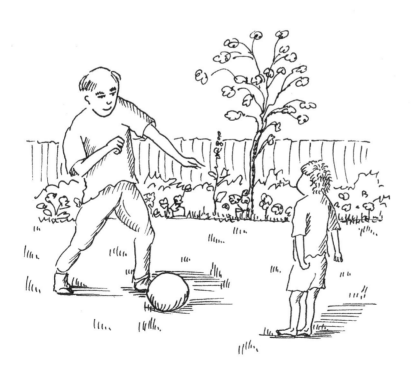

doctors and patients and between teachers and pupils. Status games are a way of bringing brief scenes alive and understand that this is how people actually behave. Read Johnstone's book and find out more; the book also includes excellent ideas for lots of different games.

Once we can understand and experience games as something we can do for fun and not turn them into battles, then we can develop them both as warm-ups and as creative techniques in themselves. We usually learn games at home as part of the playful activities of our early development. Maybe members of the group can share their experiences, both negative and positive.

Worksheet 4.1
The Prince and the Beggar

Name _____ Date _____

There are two characters: a prince and a beggar.
Sketch their costumes in the space below.

Write down a brief 'status' conversation between them –
maximum six lines.

_____

_____

_____

_____

_____

Routledge Taylor & Francis Group

Worksheet 4.2
How High Are You?

Name _____ Date _____

Draw the headdresses of people with high status and
those with low status: for example, the chef wears a tall
hat and his assistants wear shorter hats.
Military people often wear tall headdresses to
intimidate the enemy – or their inferiors.
Hats often have to be removed in the
presence of high status people.
The way we keep on our head attire or remove it
and its actual size says a lot about our status,
gender and the type of space we are in.

You can continue your drawings on the back of this sheet.

CHAPTER 5

A Little Touch of Something

MANY OF THE ADULTS WITH WHOM we work have experienced early neglect, rejection or abuse. They may well have experienced chaotic or fearful attachments, and parenting that was not 'good enough'. Early attachment is based on a physical, nurturing relationship with the mother or primary carer and it is a very playful relationship. This first 'playmate' not only fulfils the infant's physical needs of warmth, food, drink and shelter, but also is an important figure in terms of sensory development and the whole stage of Embodiment.

I have written extensively on the importance of sensory development (Jennings 2004a, 2005b) in the early life of the child. We process the world through our senses, and my concept of 'playlore' demonstrates the crucial role of our archaic sensory system in our development. The senses are physical and we learn about them in close proximity to and in physical touch from, our mothers. For people who have not had this early experience we need to find ways, through our drama work, of redressing some of the balance. Bearing in mind that many people do not like to be touched, and that many practitioners are anxious about touching people, we need to find a way that is both acceptable to the people in our groups and to ourselves.

Many staff are worried about 'health and safety', the misinterpretation of physical signals and the threat of litigation. It is not surprising that people who have been abused physically or sexually may have a negative reaction to a hand on the shoulder, however reassuring its intention.

Gerhardt in her book *Why Love Matters* (Gerhardt, 2004), is very clear about the outcomes of a lack of early nurture:

> Those who lack self-esteem and the capacity to regulate themselves may well become very self-centred adults. Without effective and well-resourced emotional systems, they cannot behave flexibly or respond to others' needs. They tend to be rather rigid, either attempting not to need others at all or needing them too much. Because they have not had enough experience of being well cared for and well regulated, their original baby needs remain active within.
> (Gerhardt, 2004)

Within the imaginative approach of a drama programme it is possible to re-experience some aspects of our early life in a more satisfying way. We can take on roles that are stronger than ourselves, or play a caring parent even though we did not have one. We can listen to stories where there are more positive outcomes and become aware of the possibility of transformation.

This type of work is challenging and at times seems without reward. For a while, people usually take only small steps forward, or two steps forward and three steps back. However, we need always to be aware of the enormous damage that many people have suffered and to understand that it will take a long time to repair or even modify.

As Cozolino so aptly writes:

> Each of us is born twice: first from our mother's body over a few hours, and again from our parents' psyche over a lifetime. If the 'second birth' does not take place or is very destructive then we will fail to thrive emotionally.
> (Cozolino, 2002)

Our brains may not develop, nor will our sensory system be intact, which in turn affects our capacity to form relationships in later life. The world is then often experienced as one fearful landscape that people need to defend against: strong defences are built to make sure that nothing comes too close. We may continue to be the terrified child who needs to cling on in desperation to anyone and everyone, or who shuns everybody, repeating patterns of early rejection.

> Many people grow older without growing up at all.
> (Garland, 2001)

Early Sensory Experience

Nurture, sensory stimulus and playfulness start before we are born the first time. Pregnant women need time to get to know their growing baby without anxieties about housing and food. The mother's emotions transmit to the unborn child, so it is important that they are positive. Love, affection, touch and sounds are also experienced in utero, and contribute to the healthy development of the unborn child. I want to repeat two important pictures from Chapter 2, because they highlight the core of what we are talking about: the playful pregnancy and the playful parental relationships.

Once we are born into the social world, we then require positive affirmation and a secure attachment with our mothers. We also need a strong relationship with both parents (even if one is unavoidably absent) in order to continue our healthy development.

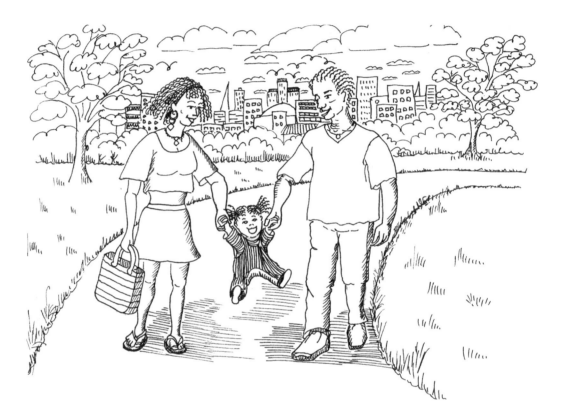

However, it is not only early experiences that can be damaging to our identity or to our sense of self. Trauma at any age disrupts our sense of identity. For example, following rape we can feel unclean and the need to keep washing ourselves: we may feel that we are permanently sullied and will never be loved. People who have had major robberies feel that their home is violated and will never be the same again. We may struggle with our identity because we did not have enough good enough parenting; we may also struggle with our identity because we have suffered an adult trauma.

Therapeutic Nurturing Experiences

How can we discover nurturing experiences that will reassure us and help us to grow rather than stay trapped in vicious cycles of addiction and mistrust? Is it possible to nurture ourselves as one way of beginning the 'repair'? How can we care for ourselves in such a way that we begin to feel more valued and more loved?

Many schools have now developed what they call nurture groups, where children meet with adult workers and have something to eat and maybe also some cuddles – this depends on the school and the experience of the staff. However, I have not yet found nurture groups for adults that will create an ambience of care and support within the therapeutic setting.

RD Laing and 'Mary Barnes'

The early work of RD Laing created some exceptional therapeutic settings, where certain people were encouraged to regress to babyhood, with baby feeding bottle and nappies, his most famous person being Mary Barnes. The story of her treatment programme has been written up extensively and is movingly portrayed in David Edgar's play *Mary Barnes* (Edgar, 1978). I well remember seeing this play when it first opened. A large group of psychoanalysts and psychotherapists were also present. They recoiled as the actress Patti Love playing Mary Barnes came on stage, naked, and dripping in faeces, and looked most uncomfortable for the rest of the evening.

In the play, Mary is encouraged to regress as far as she wants. There are feeding bottles for her instead of the stomach tubes that she has requested in order for food to be fed directly into her.

The psychiatrist in the play describes her situation.

Mary Barnes was born in 1923, feet first, without her fingernails. She couldn't suck. Her mother's pain. No milk to give. The agony inside her.

She couldn't speak. Brother came into her bedroom and tried to touch her. He was diagnosed as schizophrenic and put in a mental hospital. She converted to Catholicism.

Four years later she was diagnosed schizophrenic, put in a mental hospital. A padded cell. Discharged within a year. Returned to her career as a nurse. But underneath it all, still crazy.

But she kept herself at bay. Until she came to live in the community.
(Edgar, 1978)

This extract illustrates very well the protagonist's lack of early nurture, the abusive family and the desperate attempts to 'stay sane' until she is in an ambience that can accept her 'madness'.

Communicating Nurture and Care

We may not be able to provide a place where someone can totally regress to an infant state and re-experience better parenting. However, I am sure we can provide the elements of good parenting, both in our attitude towards people and in certain activities and resources that communicate nurture and care.

For example, much of our care is enshrined within human rights legislation, both for adults and children. I use the following topics for training and discussion. Everyone has the right:

- To feel safe at any age, which may involve protection from imagined fears as well as actual ones.

- To adequate housing, food and clothing, and not all people are in a position to provide that for themselves.
- To assistance with things they cannot manage for themselves.
- To encouragement and support, so as be as independent as possible.
- To access to the arts and their own culture.

These are the basic ingredients that we expect to find within a caring system. However, we have a very different reaction when someone is 'taken into care': appropriate homes cannot be found, there is a lack of funding and we can find ourselves in a cycle of abuse yet again.

Attachments Through the Drama Group

Basic care cannot necessarily provide the opportunities for developing 'healthy attachments' like those that we should have experienced as a child. I am proposing that the drama group is a very good place for these attachments to be modelled. The drama group is like a playground where many of the qualities and themes from child play can be developed and re-experienced in ways that are acceptable to adults. The drama group can be a nurturing playgroup where we can experiment with life as well as being sure of predictable adult support.

A person does not necessarily have to be a dramatherapist to create this model of 'nurture drama'. Nevertheless it is important to have basic understanding of attachment and the developmental needs of children and adults.

Help your group to think about what aspects of life make them feel nurtured by working through Worksheet 5.1. Help to raise people's awareness of positive and negative aspects of their lives using Worksheets 5.2 and 5.3.

The following techniques can create feelings of nurture and can be a group activity in themselves, or can be a part of other creative activities. I am still experimenting with these ideas so I could call it 'work in progress'. I always appreciate any feedback and ideas from other people.

In terms of a nurturing environment, I like many of these ideas to be a part of how I work anyway. Environments can be caring and warm rather than austere and distant. At one of the universities where I worked as a senior lecturer (the one and only time), all the staff wanted to come and visit me in my room – where I had an electric toaster, butter and blackcurrant jam!

I also had a coat that I kept hanging behind the door, together with an old briefcase with various innocuous papers in it. I always needed to know that I had a way of being 'away' without being noticed. Without people knowing where I am – just for a short time. Maybe it is a family trait, as my father hated being 'pursued' by his patients' families, so for a time he would disappear into the landscape! That is the effect that institutions have on me – I always need to know that I can exit without being noticed. I had a big smile to myself recently when the British actor Dame Judi Dench said that she always hangs her coat nearest the door when she is starting rehearsal of a new play, so that she can exit if necessary!

How can we make our work setting, even if it is an institution, more creative and welcoming? We need to be able to counter the effects of institutionalisation. I used to think that it would cease to become an issue, once the large hospitals had closed down. I then realised that there is such a thing as the 'institution of the mind', whether or not there are tangible brick walls and barbed wire.

Many play and drama techniques can be useful both with staff as well as vulnerable people. I will discuss the 'counter institution' at the end of this chapter.

The 'Soft' Environment

We do not have to spend a lot of money to create soft surroundings: for example, soft lighting can be achieved using Japanese paper shades, coloured bulbs or Chinese lanterns. Drapes of cheesecloth or soft cotton that are longer then the windows or the walls will drape in soft folds; velveteen cloths and silk scarves create textures. Plants, stones, crystals and bowls of fruit will all contribute to a nurturing environment. Make sure that allergies are checked out and that there are no food and drink rules (personally I would like to ban carbonated chemical drinks).

Think about all the senses – sight, sound, smell, taste, touch: mobiles (of the hanging variety!), candles, incense, pot-pourri, liquorice, chimes, indoor plants and a water feature. Some further ideas are provided on the following pages.

I am sure there are more nurturing exercises that you can think of, and the group itself will also have ideas. It may be that they can think of good memories amongst the negative ones, and can build on them. Encourage members of the group to bring in favourite stories, and soothing examples, such as the feel of warm towels or the smell of new-mown grass.

The whole aim is to re-learn nurturing experiences and realise that change is possible. We may even have a toy that we had when we were small. We may want to keep a scrapbook of good memories, with photographs, post cards and cuttings. Perhaps these are activities that we can develop within the group through art and craft, through music and discussion.

The Bodily Attachment

None of these exercises will help unless we are able to create the affirmation of the body, the potential for attachment through the body. It is these early physical experiences that are so essential, and if we have missed them we must find ways to re-create them. It is a paradox that through our early physical dependence we learn our independence.

Nurturing Experiences for Adults

- Self-soothing: with good quality moisturiser or baby lotion, everyone massages their own hands and wrists.

- Exercise caution if people have been sexually abused, as the texture may have unfortunate associations. You can also use almond oil as an alternative (check the strength).

- Lavender massage oil is very healing and can be used on the face as well as the hands and arms.

- Sit in a comfortable position and place your right hand on your left shoulder; gently squeeze the shoulder muscles from the neck outwards, in again and finally outwards. Repeat with the left hand on the right shoulder.

- With the middle finger of each hand, lightly massage from under the ears down to the shoulder.

- Repeat round the jaw line; massage the cheeks with several fingers.

- Place two fingers either side of the temples and make circles. Move the fingers into the hairline: there is usually a lot of tension there that needs some massage.

- Lace the fingers of both hands, place on top of the head and gently massage the scalp, forward and back.

- Do the same on the crown of the head and at the back of the head, encouraging the scalp to be flexible.

Routledge
Taylor & Francis Group

P This page may be photocopied for instructional use only. *Creative Play & Drama with Adults at Risk* © Sue Jennings 2005

Nurturing Experiences for Adults (continued)

- Place the hands at the back of the neck and move them across alternately, encouraging the muscles to relax.

- Breathe deeply, in and out, taking the same length of time for inspiration and expiration.

- Make a deep sigh and breathe out noisily (there are more breathing exercises in Chapter 6).

- Sit warmly and comfortably and drink a hot drink.

- Sit warmly and comfortably and listen to soothing music.

- Sit on cushions and cover with a blanket and listen to a soothing story.

- Curl up, feel warm and relaxed, and listen to a favourite story.

The Temiar People and Multiple Attachments

I have written extensively about my research with the Temiar peoples, and how their children become very independent and yet are breast-fed until they are five years old (Jennings, 1997). The Temiars are an interesting example of multiple attachments, where there is intense physical attachment and nurture between mother and child, with a lot of involvement by the father, but other family members are also part of the attachment circle. It seems to work! No child is left to cry, babies are fed on demand night and day, children are not hit or slapped. When tiny they are carried constantly: first on the hip, then on the back. Even five year olds carry a one year old on their backs as they play at families. And that same five year old may well be suckling at her mother's breast later that day.

As well as this powerful physical bonding, there are other ways of strengthening the parent-child relationship for the Temiars. Firstly, they believe in being linked by their naming system: when a woman is pregnant, both father and mother are called 'pregnant' as their name. Once the child is born, both parents are known by the same name: either 'parents of a boy' or 'parents of a girl'. So to make sure that one particular set of parents will answer if called, you add on the name of the child! So parents are known by the gender and name of their child.

The Temiars also believe that everyone has several souls, and at birth the head soul is the weakest and least developed. Both parents are extremely careful not to endanger the head soul of their child, who is believed to be protected by the parent's head soul until they are more independent. It means that parents are very vigilant to make sure that they protect their small children and that they both feel equally responsible.

What I learned from this was a very clear example of the importance of early physical dependence and how it creates children who are physically independent at an earlier age, when compared with their European counterparts. When we are working with adults we sometimes get irritated at their tenacity at 'holding on' – whether literally or metaphorically. In the drama group we can do plenty of 'holding on' exercises, practising trust techniques as well as those to encourage independence and resilience.

'Angry' Food and 'Soft' Food

This is a very recent idea that I have been developing in relation to nurturing experiences. We not only need the 'soft approach'; we also need ways of expressing our anger and frustrations. I have been playing with the idea that certain foods are very scrunchy: they have a real bite and we are able to gnash our teeth! A lot of contemporary food, especially fast food, is very 'pappy'; it is bland and has no texture. Many people add monosodium glutamate or very hot spices such as salsa or chilli sauce or curry – to give it a kick.

I was very surprised to learn that the UK consumes twice as many potato crisps *as the rest of Europe put together*. This really surprised me and then started me thinking. I class potato crisps as 'angry food', they are very good to munch and scrunch, and always seem amplified in a cinema! I wonder if young people are much angrier here than in other countries? Are crisps an antidote to all the other 'soft' food because they have a hot flavour – especially those with chilli, vinegar and pepperoni.

Ideas for angry food include:

- Crisps of assorted flavours – if possible those with low salt/no salt
- Rice cakes with or without sesame seeds
- Crispbreads of all kinds, but the thick rye ones crunch better
- Apples and carrots
- Peanuts and nuts of all kinds (providing there are no allergies)
- Green and red peppers, eaten raw
- Crunchy cereal: cornflakes, clusters
- Well-done toast with thick-cut marmalade

These foods contrast with soft food (which is childlike but not harmful):

- Custard made with custard powder
- Avocado
- Porridge
- Rice pudding
- Jelly

- Soft bread rolls
- Yoghurt
- Mashed potato

Both types of food can be included with lunches as part of a nurturing experience. Again, find out from the group their ideas for angry and soft food that can also be healthy. Use Worksheet 5.4 to explore their thoughts on food.

The Fear of Change

Many of the people with whom we work – both group members and staff – are terrified of change. Life has been so full of nasty surprises that they hold on to an unsatisfactory present, rather than risk change for a more fulfilling future.

Despite new research and training techniques, the ideas of empowerment, advocacy and human rights are still slow in being actualised. However, although we cannot impose change by issuing directives, we can have an inclusive approach towards our work and role model the possibilities for change. In some situations, this may be an uphill task – for example:

- A school where there is a bullying ethos amongst the staff, yet pupils are expected not bully others.
- A college that is so institutionalised that the staff boycott any event that is organised by the new principal.
- A hospital that may increase the drug regime at the weekends so that potentially more staff can have time off.
- An old peoples' home that encourages people to stay indoors, be quiet and watch television and discourages activity.

However hard we try to create democracies we are still working within very hierarchical systems. Drama-based training is one way we can help to meet some of these entrenched attitudes. Building more confident people from the beginning is the only way to bring about long-term change. The story below is a humorous example.

A Story of Empowerment

An old lady was at the checkout of the supermarket, a handful of items in her basket. As the cashier checked each item through, the old lady reminded her that the biscuits were free. 'Oh no', said the cashier, 'the price is marked on the packet'. 'I'm sorry' said the old lady, 'but it definitely says they are free. Buy two, get one free'. 'Yes' said the cashier, 'but you have only one packet so it must be paid for'. The queue is now becoming restive and people are casting their eyes up to heaven. 'Right,' said the old lady; 'I bought one packet two weeks ago, one packet a week ago, so this is my free packet'. 'But' said the cashier with exaggerated patience, 'you have to buy them all at the same time'. 'Ah' said the old lady, 'perhaps you would show me where it says that!' She left with her free packet of biscuits.

Worksheet 5.1
Feeling Good

Name _____ Date _____

Think about each thing that makes you feel good.
Is it certain types of weather? Is it certain things
you need around you? Is it a certain routine to your day?
Is it meeting certain people?

Notice how we use the word 'certain' in this context.

Write about or draw below the certainties that are
important for you to feel safe and secure.

Worksheet 5.2
The Healing Tree

Name _____ Date _____

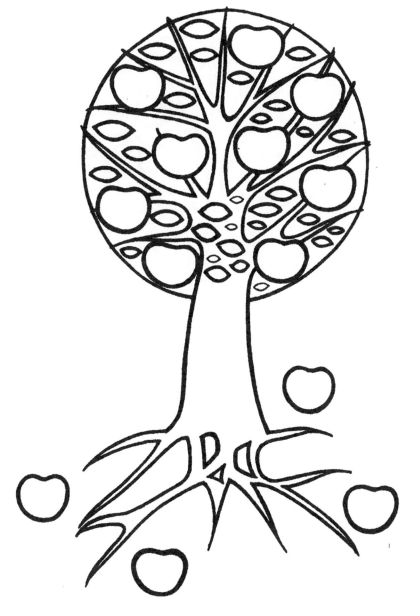

Think about your life as a tree bearing apples. Each apple represents one important aspect of your life: write the name of one aspect of your life on each one. Colour in the positive and important apples which are on the tree. Consider the fruit on the ground as aspects of your life that you have neglected: colour in those which need your attention.

Routledge
Taylor & Francis Group

P This page may be photocopied for instructional use only. *Creative Play & Drama with Adults at Risk* © Sue Jennings 2005

Worksheet S.3
The Tree of Life

Name _____ Date _____

Our senses are our deepest experience from which other things can grow and develop – especially our creativity.

Colour or paint and label the parts of the tree that belong to your life.

Routledge
Taylor & Francis Group

Worksheet 5.4
Food for Thought

Name _____ Date _____

Our food is not just important for keeping us alive,
it is also important because it looks and tastes good.
We enjoy different flavours; we meet socially for
a drink or a meal. Certain foods help to build
our brains and our nervous system.

Describe the most fantastic banquet that you would
like to attend. What would be on the menu? Who else
would be there? Where would it be held?

Write about or draw this banquet below in as much detail as
possible, and maybe use it as a theme for a drama session.

Routledge Taylor & Francis Group

P This page may be photocopied for instructional use only. *Creative Play & Drama with Adults at Risk* © Sue Jennings 2005

CHAPTER 6

A Voice for All Seasons

IN CHAPTER 5 WE FOCUSED on the importance of nurturing experiences in early life, and the idea of playful relationships and secure attachments enabling us to grow strong, confident and independent. We will now explore the importance of our voices as part of our identity, and the part they play in allowing us to express our feelings.

There are several areas that influence our voice:

- Situations where we are ridiculed
- Oppressive child-rearing where we are not allowed to speak
- Excluding child-rearing where we are not listened to
- Families where we learn half truths
- Instances where we carry the burden of guilt
- Bullying and abusive relationships
- Incidents that cause us fear and anxiety

The Effects of Fear

What better image of fear than the picture by the Norwegian painter, Munch, which is usually called *The Scream*. Everyone knows this picture; it is even moulded as a Halloween mask. No wonder thieves have gone to such lengths to steal it. There is something primal in this scream that speaks to all of us. We are not allowed to scream; we are asked to calm down and 'talk about it', but usually words cannot express these feelings. A very moving play called *Silent Scream*, by Andy Hickson (2002), is touring schools and colleges. The play is about bullying and its damaging effects. Pupils then take part in workshops on 'finding your voice': finding the voice that will tell, and not just stay as a silent scream.

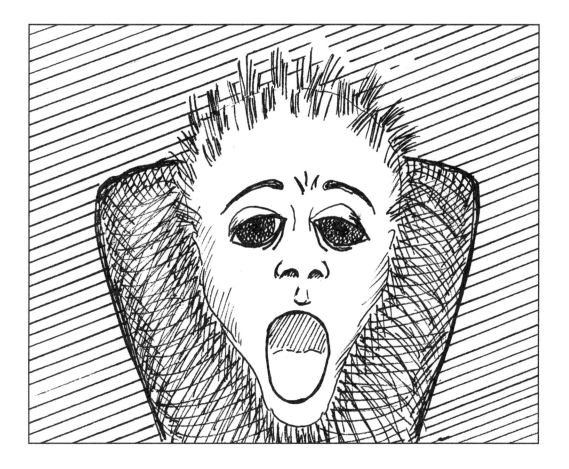

We notice that children who are not allowed a voice, who have not been listened to or who have been made fun of, will either go silent or will only shout. It is either 'all inside' or 'all outside'. The child who goes silent has everything under control and is self-contained; he or she is often thought to be 'good'. However, other indicators can appear, such as insomnia, or perpetual throat infections or headaches. Keeping it all in can affect other parts of the body and result in pain and tension: the body is crying in other ways.

The child who resorts to 'total shout' gradually loses all sense of self and so shouts louder. All boundaries become broken and very often there is a total tantrum: the child throws him – or herself on the floor, absolutely 'beside himself'. Unfortunately I also encounter parents who think this is very funny and will not intervene. It becomes a sort of entertainment.

Observing the Emotions of Others

We can also see the extreme emotions of others on television. Viewing such emotions is one of the reasons why people watch cookery programmes, chat shows, 'get me out' shows, 'real' soaps, hellish neighbours and so called 'help programmes'. When people get angry, the audience cheers – just as in Ancient Rome, where the audiences were entertained by gladiators trying to defend themselves against wild animals.

It is true that we have professional actors whose job it is to portray the human condition. However, the expression of strong emotions is no longer the sole province of the actor: so called 'ordinary people' are invited to perform them instead! The out-of-control language and voices are also entering the domains of advertising: in the UK we are asked to yell for phone numbers or to shout to clean our clothes or grab a bag of crisps. Yet the more we shout, the less we can hear anyone else.

> Children and adults need to be heard and to know that they are listened to, with respect and patience.
> (Jennings, 2004e)

> We need to be able to express our own needs and ideas without fear of ridicule or being shouted down.
> (Jennings, 2004b)

Lies and Half-truths

Unfortunately there is still the belief that children should not be told what is going on in the family, so they pick up innuendoes and half-truths. They can feel excluded and betrayed, and then very angry when they learn the truth in later life. Many of our damaged adults are the victims of a conspiracy of silence about crucial facts or events in their early family history, which may include:

- Member(s) of the family are abusers.
- The criminal history of a relative.
- Adoption by new parents.
- A medical history involving serious illness: physical and/or mental.
- The death of a sibling.
- Abuse by a parent or sibling.
- Situations that are considered 'failures', such as redundancy or bankruptcy.

The story of *The Railway Children* by E Nesbit is a poignant example of a family secret that is kept from children for some time, and which requires the mother to 'keep up appearances'.

Discovering my True Voice

The following exercises will help us to discover our authentic voice and to build up our confidence. All our drama work will help us grow and expand, but our voices play a special part in our development.

The Voice Chart
(the outside voices)

- What are the different voices that you can recall from your own life? Maybe people in your own childhood had distinctive voices, maybe positive, maybe negative.

- Put your own name in the centre of a piece of paper: draw a circle around it, and then a series of circles round edge. Put the name of the person and the quality of the voice you remember in each circle.

- What were/are these voices saying to you? Consider whether each voice is invasive or critical? Or does it communicate support or affirmation?

- What messages did you get from members of your family, especially your parents? Do you want to change those that are 'inside your head'?

- Which of the voices from the outside, from other people, do you appreciate? What is the tone of the voice? (See Worksheet 6.1).

- Do you have voice memories that may not be critical but the sound is harsh, grating or 'like a fish wife'?

- Similarly, do you recall voices that sound warm, clear or firm?

- Think of as many words as you can to describe the qualities of voices: both positive and negative.

- Think about the quality of voice that you would like to acquire.

Authentic Voice
(the inside voices)

- How can we find our authentic voice – the one that belongs to us?

- Practise listening to your own voice. If you would like to change it, decide how.

- If there are complex reasons that have influenced your voice, make sure you spend time in understanding them. Remember that they come from the outside, not the inside. They may have made you fearful or angry or burdened.

- Play with your voice – saying different things in different ways, saying them fast and saying them slow, saying them loud and saying them soft.

- Remember the breathing exercises we have already learned and breathe in enough breath to keep your voice strong.

- From the voice map Worksheets (6.1 to 6.3), what qualities of voice would you like to acquire. Do you need strength, variety, firmness, clarity or warmth?

- Play with those qualities, think of characters in films or plays that have voices you find attractive. Are there personalities on television, such as newsreaders, whose voices you like?

Routledge
Taylor & Francis Group

Authentic Voice (the inside voices) (continued)

- When working on improvisation, theatre scenes or storytelling, try out different types of voice and allow yourself to take on new qualities.

- Keep a voice diary about your own voice and its changes, and your new sensibility to the sounds of the voices around you.

Saying No!
(and meaning it)

- It is your right to be able to speak for yourself and be heard.

- It is your right to have choices about things you wish to do and to have your choice respected.

- Sometimes our voice is not heard amongst the clamour. If all else fails, hold up a hand on a stick to make sure you are noticed!

- Were you allowed to speak for yourself as a child? And were you heard? Maybe there were other demands within the family from people that were ill or several younger siblings.

- Did you go to a school where you were encouraged to speak? Or was speaking only for the quick and clever pupils? Was it a question of 'Sit down and shut up', 'Heads down and get on with your work', 'Who will be the first with the answer?' or 'Which clever person can tell me *now?*'

- Were you so disenchanted with family or school that you just 'switched off' so you did not hear anything?

- Did you make a decision that to switch off was at least one decision that you could make for yourself?

- Write down all the things you want to say 'no' to from the past: try to find a way to let go of them because they are in the past.

Routledge Taylor & Francis Group

Saying No! (and meaning it) (continued)

- Write down all the things you want to say 'no' to in the present. Which are the most important?

- Create a role-play where you can practise saying 'no'. Try it out with different people and get their feedback.

- Write a tough poem about saying 'no'. Make sure that it really expresses your feelings.

- Cut out words from newspapers to create a picture that says 'no'.

- Remember that you also need to communicate saying 'no' with your body: for example, stand your ground and stay while other people try to 'push you around'.

- Hold hands with a partner and don't allow yourself to be pulled across the room. If there is not enough space for this, try 'arm wrestling', Chinese style.

- Think of all the bodily expressions that communicate feelings: for example we can 'stay our ground', 'we can elbow our way in', 'we can stick our nose in', 'we can put our best step forward' – there are many, many more.

- Think of a cause that you feel strongly about. Write a short speech about it and deliver your speech. Think of something specific that you want stopped (that you want to say 'No' to).

- Then try turning your idea around and approaching it in a different way. Rather than stopping something, is

Saying No! (and meaning it) (continued)

there another thing that you could encourage? Notice how your voice changes when you are able to support something in contrast to when you want to stop something.

- Consider the following pictures (on Worksheet 6.3). Copy the expressions, say something and see what sort of voice is coming out. What sort of character might have a voice like this?

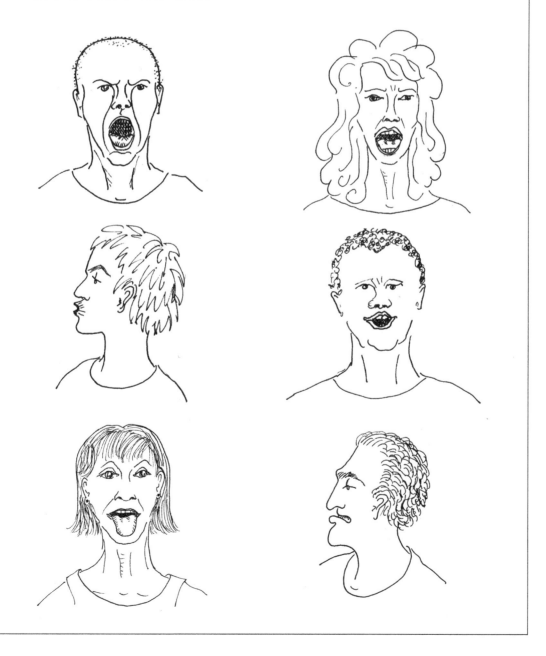

Routledge
Taylor & Francis Group

Voice Warm-ups and Development

- Physical warm up to music – letting go of tension – check especially that neck, jaw and shoulders are not tense.

- Practise sighing and yawning alternately.

- Breathe in and expand your ribcage and slowly breathe out again.

- Breathe in and vocalise the vowel sound 'ahhhh' as you breathe out.

- Repeat with the sound 'oooh'.

- Loosen up your tongue and lips by repeating the consonants:

    'b', 'd', 'g' and 'p', 't', 'k'.

- Try these tongue twisters: 'Peter Piper picked a peck of pickled peppers' or 'Sally sells seashells on the seashore'. Repeat each one six times without stumbling.

- Choose a vowel sound and 'throw it' with your voice across the room to another person – make the sound and quite literally throw it with your hand. It is then caught by your partner and then thrown back, either the same sound or another one.

Routledge
Taylor & Francis Group

P This page may be photocopied for instructional use only. Creative Play & Drama with Adults at Risk © Sue Jennings 2005

Voice Warm-ups and Development (continued)

- Imagine you are on top of a mountain and you want to communicate something across the valley; make your voice strong without shouting and decide what this important thing is you have to say. Create a strong voice and call!

- Imagine you are in a place where you cannot raise your voice, how quietly can you speak and still be understood?

- Is it possible to express a strong feeling by mouthing the words with no sound at all? What happens to the rest of your body? And your face muscles?

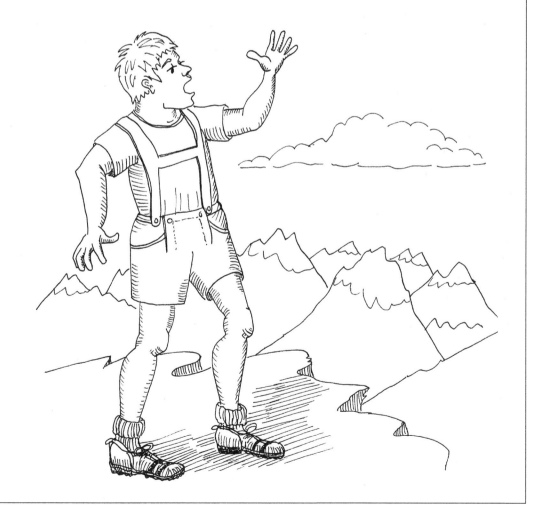

Routledge
Taylor & Francis Group

P

Voice Triangles

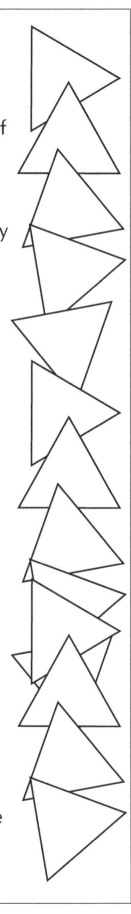

One

- In groups of three create a scene with an angry voice, a scared voice and a calm voice. Decide who the people are. Notice if there is an alliance between the scared voice and the calm voice.

- Repeat the exercise realising that the angry voice may also be scared, and have a different way of covering it up.

- Discuss why each voice might have developed and see if it depends on your understanding of the character and their 'authenticity'.

Two

- Develop a triangle with others of three phrases from your childhood that you can recall. Were these phrases in conflict?

- Take it in turns so that all members of the group can explore their phrases.

- Are there voices and phrases that are similar between different groups and individuals?

- Play with the idea of an echo where phrases that are common to the group are stated strongly and then echoed several

Routledge
Taylor & Francis Group

P

times, gradually dying away; before if finishes another phrase comes in, and echoes.

Three

- Take three phrases from legends, proverbs or sayings and create a voice scene where they are echoed to each other.

- Check out whether there are 'sayings' from your childhood that you could play with too, such as 'Little girls are seen and not heard'.

- Share the voice scenes with the group and feed back experiences.

- Choose the most powerful voices and phrases and create a 'chorus' that speaks before the characters speak.

- Create a chorus that speaks what the character is feeling inside but not saying; so the character speaks and their internal voice is speaking under the words, or following on from their words.

- Create one voice that is like a conscience, that speaks an 'aside' to what ever the character is saying.

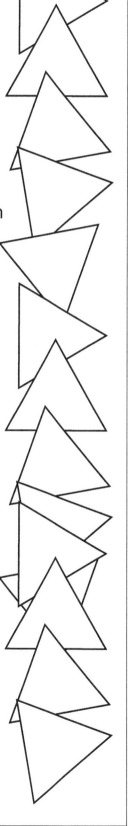

Routledge
Taylor & Francis Group

P

Voice Triangles
(continued)

Four

- Take three lines from a poem, a Shakespeare play or a myth. These lines must form the 'core' of something really important; explore them in groups of three. Everyone can learn three lines, or it could be just one line if you have one each. Explore different ways of saying them.

- What gestures go with these phrases? Are they expressed standing up or sitting down? Would you have a costume that could get in the way of saying these lines?

- Do you have to carry a prop in relation to these lines? Will it emphasise the phrases or the meaning, establish your authority or add to your character?

- How much can be established through your voice rather than through props and costumes? Remember: a prop can be overused as a prop to hold you up, rather than one of the *properties* that are necessary for the character.

- Notice that your understanding of the words or the poem continues to deepen with the amount of time you spend exploring through your voice. My voice can be the key to my heart!

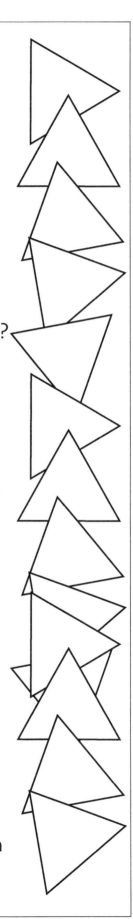

I tell all the people I work with:

> The deeper we explore and develop our voices, the deeper we can
> understand ourselves, and the drama of our lives.

and also:

> Remember the call of the wild? The call of the forest? The howl of the wolf
> on the mountain? The earthy sound of the music of Pan?
> It is real sound and gets deep into our bones.

> Our first task is to recover the call of the heart.
> (Newham, 1999)

Indigenous Calling

Newham (1999) wrote about remembering what it means 'to call'; he describes it as the indigenous call of people, whatever their culture:

> When the Muslim muezzin calls the people to prayer from the tower –
> this is calling. When the Quaquali singer reaches the crescendo of his epic
> song or the Welsh shepherd instructs his dog on the other side of the field –
> this is calling. When the railroad builders and cotton pickers projected
> their voices over huge distances or when the American cowboys
> yodelled from their ranch – this was calling.
> (Newham, 1999)

Go back to the picture of the man on the mountain and think about yourself and the idea of 'calling'. What raw and natural sound can you allow yourself to express that does not have all the layers of your fear and anger? Work through this with the group using Worksheet 6.4.

Perhaps we are beginning to understand the powerhouse that can be our voice if we allow it. We do not need to be scared or timid or out of control. Our voice is a very finely tuned instrument that belongs to our soul. It is sad if we poison it with toxins or stress or misuse.

Healthy voices now calling!

Worksheet 6.1
The Voice Map – Many Voices

Name _____ Date _____

Create a map of all the voices that you hear in your life,
past and present.

Choose colours that represent the different feelings and, if
possible, write a key to indicate the people to whom these
voices belong.

Compare maps 6.1 and 6.2 and see which
voices you have taken from others.
Maybe some of your voices are the opposite
of ones that you hear?

Routledge
Taylor & Francis Group

P This page may be photocopied for instructional use only. *Creative Play & Drama with Adults at Risk* © Sue Jennings 2005

Worksheet 6.2
The Voice Map - Your Voice

Name _____ Date _____

Create a 'voice map' of all the different voices that you use – colour different areas to indicate the feelings behind the voices. Link the colours with the feelings: some people would say, for example, that red is an angry colour.

Worksheet 6.3
The Voice Map – Voice Collage

Name _____ Date _____

Materials needed: old newspapers and magazines, as much variety as possible; glue, scissors and stout paper or card.

Cut out as many headlines as you want that indicate different voices. Then create a small collage, either on this sheet or – preferably – on a larger piece of paper.
For example: 'The prime minister remained silent';
'"Stop!" Shouted the referee'.
Make a voice 'collage', and colour it too if you wish.

Share the collage with the group; using the style of voice that you think is appropriate. These themes can also be used and developed for improvisation.

Routledge Taylor & Francis Group

Worksheet 6.4
Calling, Calling!

Name _____ Date _____

Look at the picture of the man on the mountain and think about yourself and the idea of 'calling'. What raw and natural sound can you allow yourself to express that does not include all the layers of your fear and anger?

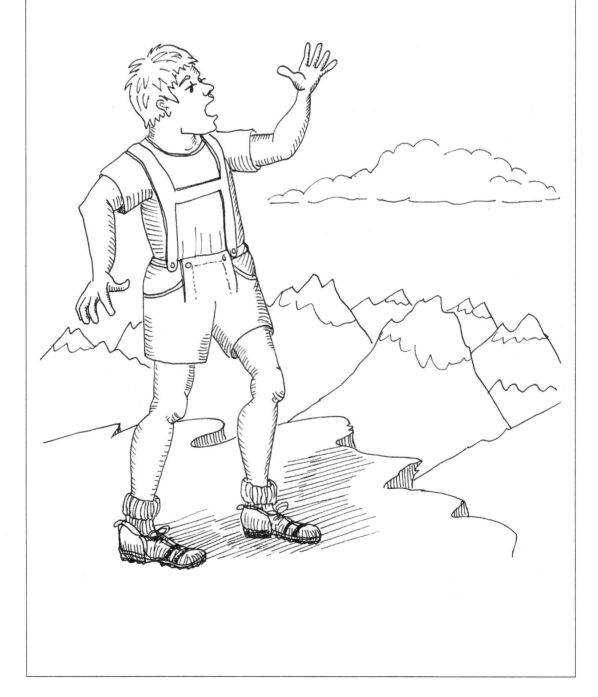

CHAPTER 7

Bring on the Clowns

AN IMPORTANT FEATURE of 'dramatic reality' is that we have permission to play, to try things out and experiment without fear of ridicule. We can explore new roles and scenes with the phrase 'What would happen if?' without others interpreting our expressions or explaining our motives.

The Products of Playfulness: an Example

In dramatic reality we can be playful without having to 'clown around'. For example, a disabled member of one of the drama groups got very 'stuck' in playing the little girl in all her interactions. She rarely listened to what was being said and if the attention was not focused on her she would switch off or talk over what other people were saying. Because she had a lot of affirmation from her carers in relation to independent living, taking time with her health and beauty and owning a wardrobe with plenty of choices and bright colours, she seemed to have got stuck in that role and had trouble moving on. She was getting plenty of 'nurture' but did not have the support to move on from what was becoming a cosy cocoon.

She needed help in making a transition into group interactions from her individual preoccupations. As a member of the group she had to learn to wait her turn and communicate to the group as a whole. She needed to learn about risk taking and about being adventurous in creative ways. She needed new challenges, and the group provided her with many challenges.

She learned new creative techniques, which included circle dancing, sword fighting, group chants, drumming and clowning. Some of these activities were for pairs and some for the whole group. Previously she allowed everyone else to clear up: she is now expected to help pack away the equipment. Now she has innovatory ideas to contribute to the group.

As a result she rang her carers and reported enthusiastically on how much fun she was having in the group, rather than everything being centred on her immediate personal needs. There were other people in the group who were more disabled than herself who looked out for her. She was beginning to take risks and loved every minute of it. This included the introduction of clown workshops to the 'special needs' groups as well as the training groups.

Clown Workshops

The introduction of the clown workshops in several of the groups I am involved with has been a very important development. There are several people who have been trained as 'sacred clowns' and they have particular routines of exercises that are helpful in encouraging the community of the groups, as well as building confidence and communication. I use the phrase the 'community of the groups' in a similar way as in the 'olden days' we would refer to the 'family of the theatre'. Everyone would look out for everyone else, and if someone were out of work then others would help out. Younger members of the profession would care for actors who became ill or elderly, even if work was not plentiful for anyone. In the theatre there has always been some sense of a community which by its very nature is out of the ordinary: actors work antisocial hours compared with everyone else; they have to move around a lot; they do jobs that make enormous emotional demands on them.

There is an important ingredient here: actors have to 'step into the void', not knowing what audience will be in and whether they will be heard or understood or whether the play will be appreciated or panned. I read Joe Simpson's book *Touching the Void* (Simpson, 1998) and was very moved by his account of being left to die on Mount Everest. I recommend his story to everyone. It is quite scary for the people in our groups to step into the unknown, and allow themselves to take risks. However, with our support you will be surprised, as the story of the disabled young woman above illustrates.

Basic Clowning
Exercises

- Create a circle, hold hands and sway all together, first one way and another; be careful with your balance.

- Stay in the same circle and experiment with swaying in different directions.

- Stay in the circle but stop holding hands. Each person tries to sit on the floor, one at a time. If two people sit down together, the whole group has to start again. People soon start to be more observant of everyone in the group, once they have re-started several times.

- Once everyone is sitting, try to stand up one at a time. The same rule applies: back to the beginning if two stand up together!

- Everyone holds on to a smooth rope, close your eyes and people can lead others slowly and carefully by gently pulling on the rope. This is a trust exercise where everyone needs to be highly tuned to the non-verbal communication of others.

- Hold the rope in a line and someone in the middle leads the group.

- Choose a partner (make sure there are even numbers in the group, otherwise you will either need to take a partner or allow one person to stay out each time). One person closes their eyes and the other person leads them on a 'blind walk'. Place either two hands on the shoulder, one hand on the shoulder or to be really risky put one finger on the shoulder!

Routledge
Taylor & Francis Group

P This page may be photocopied for instructional use only. *Creative Play & Drama with Adults at Risk* © Sue Jennings 2005

Basic Clowning Exercises (continued)

- Try the exercise again and see if people can tolerate not speaking and just communicating through the touch. You will observe that people will initially put their hands in front of them in case they bump into something. The people leading need to know it's not a jokey exercise.

- If people adapt to the mutual trust you can start to use variations such as: don't just walk round the room but explore different textures on the way; explore different levels.

- As you draw the exercise to a close, instruct the people being led, 'Before you open your eyes, tell your partner whereabouts in the room you are and where everyone else is', or, 'Before you open your eyes tell your partner whether they are taller or shorter than you and what are they wearing'.

- If group members are really confident, while one half have their eyes closed, signal the others to change with each other, and see if their partner notices – usually they don't!

- If group members are adventurous, one could lead two people with their eyes closed.

- Find ways to extend your movement so that it is larger than life – go beyond your body boundaries making enormous strides and extended swinging of the arms, and feel you are as tall as a giant.

Basic Clowning Exercises (continued)

- Write your name very large in the air.

- Write an enormous letter or number and your partner has to guess what it is.

- With your partner make patterns of large circles and lines, if you can, to a variety of different pieces of music.

- Use brightly coloured ribbons on the end of sticks: either tie them on or tack brass rings on the end. Swirl the ribbons above your head and make patterns in the air. Make circles close to the floor and other people can jump through them. You can also use long scarves made of soft material and use them in similar ways.

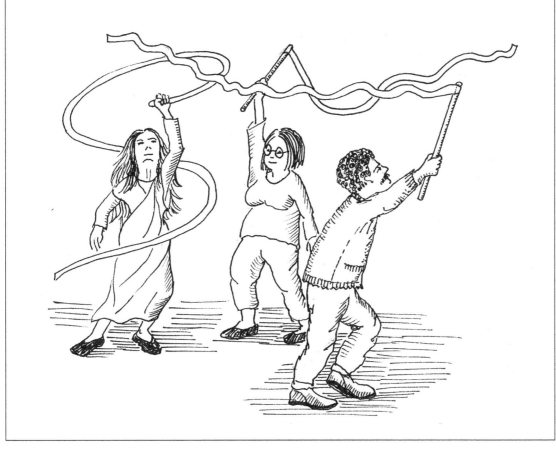

Routledge
Taylor & Francis Group

P

All the Basic Clowning Exercises can be used for general warm-ups and not just for clown workshops. They engender collaboration, support, trust, cooperation, risk taking, creativity and humour. Most of the exercises can be done to music: it should have a firm steady beat and rhythm, not too fast, to stimulate energy. Your selection might include brass band marches, circus music, African drumming, overtures to operas and ballets, or traditional jazz.

Many clowns have their own clown puppet mounted on a stick (a Punchinello); they will talk with the puppet and answer themselves, and allow them to talk to other people – that way they do not have to take responsibility for what they might say!

Props and Further Activities

- Have some clown noses, large bow ties and an assortment of hats available.

- Use Worksheets 7.1 and 7.2 to help you think about different types of clown.

- Walk round the room with your toes turned out and your arms on your hips: add your nose, bow tie and hat.

- Play with different gestures for your hands and positions for your head.

- Put on some expansive music and have some fun improvising a clown opera, ballet or ice-skating scene. Stay with the music long enough to get really into your clown character.

- Try different hats and maybe choose a prop as your clown identity is emerging.

- Remember that every clown is an individual; each one's personality and make-up is unique.

- Allow yourself to have ownership of your clown personality.

- To the song 'Puppet on a String', move as a clown puppet.

Routledge
Taylor & Francis Group

Props and Further Activities (continued)

- Put on some music from another culture: maybe Chinese ballet, African drumming or Aborigine rhythms. Dance in your character and feel that you own it physically.

- Link arms with two others and create a clog dance together.

- Create a comic sequence that incorporates dance and mime and a simple trick.

- Pretend that you are juggling with imaginary juggling balls. (Some group members may want to acquire juggling skills, which are excellent for concentration and coordination.)

- Create a juggling sequence with a partner. Remember: if you maintain hand-eye co-ordination, and your eyes follow the imaginary ball, you will be convincing.

- Blow up a balloon and clown with it and then burst it.

- Have a clown fight with another clown using balloons.

- Play with a very large strong balloon or ball: sit on it, fall off it and chase it, for example.

- Tie a strong balloon to a stick and arrange a mock fight with another clown. (Morris dancers in the UK have a comic character fighting with a 'bladder'.)

Props and Further Activities (continued)

- Create a scene where a clown has a pet dog, who perhaps trips you up.

- Clowns usually have items that are either very small or enormous – find a way to use something that is extreme in size.

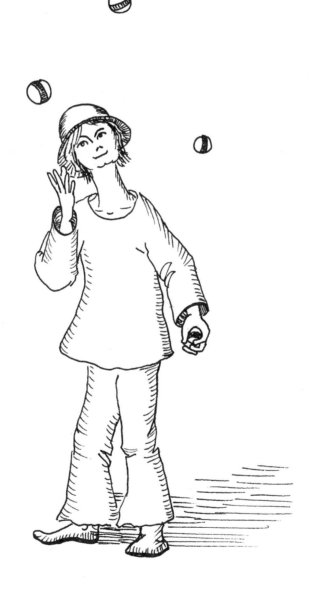

Routledge
Taylor & Francis Group

P

Clowning as a Relief From Tension

If we look at serious stories and plays there is almost always a clown figure that reduces the tension before it builds up again. The tension in a major tragedy cannot be sustained for the whole story and the clown characters break up this anticipation, allowing the audience 'off the hook' for a few moments, before it starts to build up again

Hamlet

In *Hamlet* the main clown characters are the two grave-diggers at Ophelia's funeral, and it is paradoxical that this funeral is so tragic. Her death sears into our feelings as we see her go crazy after the sudden death of her father. She falls into the river, her clothes fill up with water and she drowns. In the extract below, the queen sets the scene.

> There is a willow grows aslant a brook,
> That shows his hoar leaves in the glassy stream.
> There with fantastic garments did she come,
> Of crow-flowers, nettles, daisies, and long purples,
> That liberal shepherds give a grosser name
> But our cold maids do dead men's fingers call them.
> There, on the pendant boughs her coronet weeds
> Clambering to hang, an envious sliver broke,
> When down with her weedy trophies, and herself,
> Fell in the weeping brook. Her clothes spread wide,
> And, mermaid-like, awhile they bore her up;
> Which time, she chaunted snatches of old tunes,
> As one incapable of her own distress.
> (Shakespeare, *Hamlet,* 4, vii, 92–103)

This is almost the end of the scene as the queen is telling her new husband Claudius, and Ophelia's brother, Laertes, the circumstances of her death.

The next scene immediately takes us into the clown grave-diggers: the stage instruction actually says 'Enter two clowns, with spades and mattocks' and the location is 'A Churchyard'.

They start discussing whether Ophelia is to be allowed a Christian burial as there is talk that she killed herself. The first clown then 'proves' that she did not kill herself, as follows.

> Give me leave. Here lies the water – good. Here stands the man – good. If the man go to this water and drown himself, it is, will he nill he, he goes, mark you that. But if the water come to him and drown him, he drowns not himself. Argal, he that is not guilty of his own death, shortens not his own life.
> (Shakespeare, *Hamlet,* 5, i, 134–138)

If you read the speech again it is obvious that the grave-digger is using something, maybe stones, to illustrate his story – what we would call a 'sculpt'. Dramatherapists always used to think that they invented sculpting, but Shakespeare already had it as a device; it also occurs in *Two Gentlemen of Verona*.

The scene continues with a lot of banter between the two characters, including lighthearted references to the length of time it takes corpses to decay. The main digger is singing as he digs and Hamlet enters with Horatio.

> Has this fellow no feeling of his business that he sings at grave-making?
> (Shakespeare, *Hamlet,* 5, i, 65)

The banter between the grave-digger and Hamlet slowly gets more serious, and then the funeral begins. The clowns have lightened the mood and then there is a transition before the tragedy takes hold of us once more. Hamlet tries to reconcile himself to Ophelia's brother Laertes but there is a fight actually *in* the grave.

You could use the example from *Hamlet* quoted above to have a discussion about the role of humour in grief and tragedy. Some would have us believe that such laughter is avoidance or a defence mechanism. I am not sure of the difference. A clown's laughter is close to tears anyway and sometimes we laugh and cry at the same time. The sensations can be very similar as we laugh until the tears roll down our cheeks, or we cry and howl and then it turns to laughter.

Perhaps these emotions of tears and joy are not as far apart as we might think. Look up the work of different clowns such as Grimaldi, Joey and Patch Adams, and see how they can enhance your understanding of clowns and their work.

Circus Ideas

In groups I have worked with in the past I have taken the analogy of the circus and let participants explore different ideas such as:

- walking the tightrope
- juggling their lives
- cracking the whip
- no safety net
- a caged lion
- a performing seal

The results were very moving as people realised that many such phrases applied to their own situations. We kept the metaphor of the circus and explored within the roles.

With another group I explored the idea of 'clowning around' through games and scenes. We then painted masks for three clowns:

- the angry clown
- the sad clown
- the happy clown

Clowns and Jester Sticks

- Make a Punchinello puppet as similar to yourself as possible and use it as your jester stick.

- Let the puppet wear clothes like yours and have a bow tie or make-up that mirrors your own.

- Use Worksheet 7.3 to draw the puppet and then create a sequence where you and your jester stick ask each other questions about what you will do.

- Write the story of your clown puppet and its relationship with you.

- Plan a scene where the puppet takes control over its owner.

- Create a scene with several puppets together.

- Create time and space where each of the clown puppets can introduce themselves to the group and the group can ask questions: answer them as the puppet, not as yourself.

- Share the experiences 'out of role' – as both puppet and clown with the group.

- Think of ways you can extend this work and develop more skills.

Routledge
Taylor & Francis Group

P This page may be photocopied for instructional use only. *Creative Play & Drama with Adults at Risk* © Sue Jennings 2005

Once people had created their masks (see Worksheet 7.3) and stood back and gazed at them, there were some very powerful feelings. Many people felt that they had been set up to play the clown from an early age; sometimes it was the only way to be noticed, or a way of avoiding being bullied. This resulted in very deep feelings being acknowledged behind the clowning around. As we know, clowns can very often be unhappy people; but in my experience, people who clown around are very often angry, too. In this particular workshop most of the participants expressed some previously unacknowledged fury, which needed to be addressed over a period of several weeks. Never underestimate the powerful dynamic of any drama work, even when you are working with humour. The clown especially can unleash all kinds of feelings, but for the most part it is a good idea to keep the feelings within the character and the role. We shall learn more about these skills in Chapters 9 and 10.

Other Kinds of Masks

I have left this section until last because it is a particular favourite of mine. I use a lot of masks and most of the time we make them together in the group. We either use a paper plate as a base and build onto it, or we use a lightweight plastic mask and paint it or stick things to it, such as feathers.

Choosing and Designing Masks

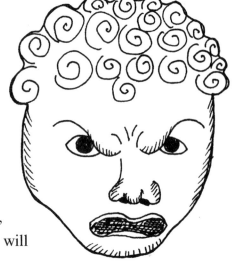

Many groups will be very inventive with their masks and wish to make use of a wider range of materials and start from scratch. However, it is important that you all decide on a theme, story or play that the masks relate to.

You may decide to show pictures of various masks to act as a stimulus, together with many different faces. This will encourage discussion of the difference between a mask and a face. People often have very definite ideas about a mask they would like to make. One way of maximising choice is to propose that each person can choose his or her own character from the story and make that character's mask. In one forensic group I gave this choice in relation to *A Midsummer Night's Dream* and almost every person chose a character that is cruel to women. After six months they chose another character with a more diverse range.

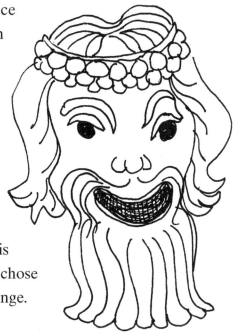

Practicalities

It is important to remember that masks need to be comfortable: people need to be able to breathe adequately or they will hyperventilate, and they need to be able to see clearly! If you have any doubts, work with small masks to start with, the type that highwaymen were supposed to don. They can have extra decoration, but the important thing is that they do not cover the nose

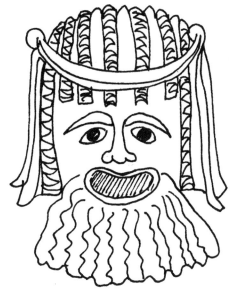

and mouth and the eyes are big enough to see through. In *Dramatherapy with Families, Groups and Individuals* (Jennings, 1990) there is a detailed description of what I call the 'mask progression'. You can start with the mask on a stick that is held in front of the face and work right through to the whole head mask.

The mask drawings shown here can be enlarged on the photocopier, stuck onto card and then coloured, or they can be used as ideas for building different masks – maybe out of papier-mâché or plaster of Paris bandage.

Please note

Great care must be taken with both these media. Some people have allergic reactions and other people feel claustrophobic if a mask is made of their faces. So you can find a polystyrene/Styrofoam head used in hat displays you can make any mask you wish!

If you are using masks for the first time, invite people to make a collage of faces of many different types or provide lots of postcards for people to look at. You may indeed want to start with puppets instead of masks as people become more relaxed about 'talking through' another image.

Worksheet 7.1
Clown Heads

Name _____ Date _____

Look at the four clown heads below and choose one to explore. What type of clown do you think each one is? Describe their tricks and jokes, and create a short scene that it could perform.

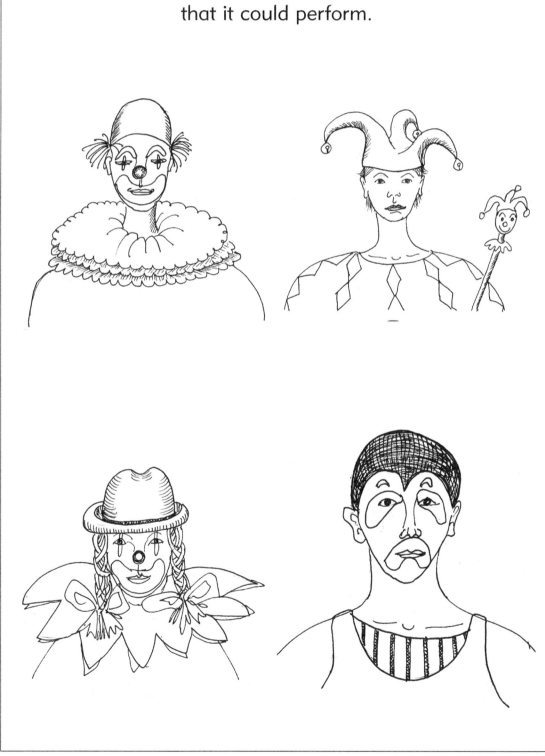

Routledge
Taylor & Francis Group

P

Worksheet 7.2
Clown Puppets

Name _____ Date _____

Draw a picture of your clown-puppet or a puppet that you would like to make. Show as much detail of the face as you can and then any clothes or props it might have.

Now write a short story about the puppet,
which starts as follows.

My name is _____

_____

_____

_____

_____

_____

You can continue your story on the back of this sheet.

Routledge
Taylor & Francis Group

P

Worksheet 7.3
Clown Feelings

Name _____ Date _____

What are the most important colours for you in expressing your clown's feelings? Is your clown mainly angry, sad or happy? Colour your clown's face with the colours you want to use to express this feeling.

My Clown Face

Write a short description of your clown below, using the first person.

My name is _____

_____

_____

_____

_____

_____

You can continue your story on the back of this sheet.

CHAPTER 8

Creative Playing Between Adults and Children

IN EARLIER CHAPTERS WE HAVE TALKED about playful relationships between adults and children, and the importance of dramatic play on our own development. In this chapter we shall examine the whole idea of the mutual benefits for adults and children of playing theatre together.

Children will cast us in many different roles in their dramatic play: sometimes they want a witness and at other times a performer; we may have to help with costumes and props, or be an arbiter regarding the time and the space. Sometimes we initiate the playing ourselves and sometimes it will come from the children. However, we cannot impose dramatic play on a child. Playing emerges in its several stages and can be endorsed and supported by adults.

> There will develop a kind of mutuality through the playing which can be pleasurable for everyone.

> The more we can play, the more we can repair some of the damage caused by the fact we were unable to play as a child.

If we did not ourselves play as children, it is possible for us to play anew through and with our own children, or the children of friends and relatives. Young children will teach us how to play and often make the most sophisticated teachers! Children can teach us about creativity, spontaneity and improvisation. Most of the exercises in this chapter can be played with children as well as adults, and children and adults can also participate together.

The following are some ideas for activities that focus on the freeing of the creative aspect of ourselves through improvisation in its many forms.

- Allow the 'breaking of rules' in order to discover a creative impulse: for example, experiment with a dramatic scene as if it is funny; read out a recipe as if it were a prison sentence.
- Let one person be a 'machine' and the other person operate it.
- Create a group machine with everyone in the group, with one inventor who constructs it.
- Invent a new machine that has never existed before and convince everyone else to buy it.
- Invent a modern version of something traditional from the kitchen.
- Create a mechanical robot that will do something to make life easier – one person builds it using another person as raw material.

Improvisation

Improvisation in dramatic play is like a 'stream of consciousness' that happens in the moment, rather than the planned drama of a scene or a text. There may be a fairly loose narrative that is made up as you go along, but it does not have to 'make sense' in the adult notion of a 'logical progression'.

The importance of improvisation is that:

- It can develop our brains to make new associations
- It can free us from stereotyped responses
- It can lead to new creative ideas
- It can help us practise real life situations

Many drama teachers and theatre directors use improvisation as a means of exploring a character, situation or text before starting work on the project or production itself.

Improvisation is like a form of 'brainstorming' in action. It is something that you do rather than talk about: it can use words or be completely non-verbal.

We can use improvisation to explore real life situations in order to find a solution, or we can use creative ideas to develop our artistic forms and structures. The skill of improvisation can be used in all aspects of our work and home: it is a way of being playful and not determining the outcome. It is very useful when we are in strange situations or if we have to think on our feet or stand in for someone. It is also useful at occasions such as weddings when we are asked 'to say a few words'.

As adults we may feel stiff, stupid or silly improvising, but if we take time to observe how young children improvise (together or alone, in the garden or in the school playground) we can be inspired! If children are allowed to play 'naturally' they will play with whatever is at hand: old boxes, scraps of material, string and newspapers. They invent stories and plays and a range of characters. However, it is important to recognise the improvisation in this playing – it is not scripted beforehand.

Encouraging Creativity and Spontaneity

What is the child thinking about who drew this picture?

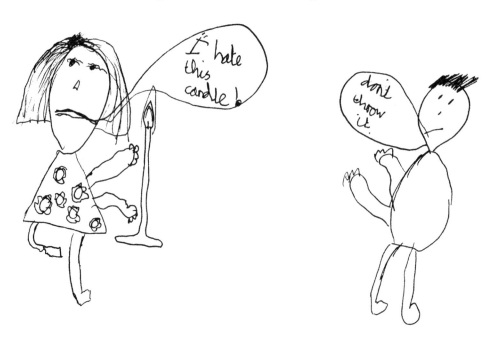

Many teachers discourage children's creativity and spontaneity, and prefer conformity. Keith Johnstone writes:

> Most schools encourage children to be *unimaginative*. The research so far shows that imaginative children are disliked by their teachers. Imagination is as effortless as perception, unless we think it might be 'wrong', which is what our education encourages us to believe. Then we experience ourselves as 'imagining', as 'thinking up an idea', but what we are really doing is faking up the sort of imagination we think we ought to have,
>
> (Johnstone,1981)

Many people who are encouraged to attend a drama group are scared of being laughed at by 'making fools of themselves'; or they feel that they will be criticised for not 'getting it right'. They may well have been squashed as children when they offered creative ideas in class or perhaps they came from a home where formal learning was imposed and 'playing' was seen as a waste of time. We talk about 'real work' and 'real study' as if it is nothing to do with play. We need to remind ourselves that 'learning though playing' is the most efficient way of both understanding and retaining what we have learned. Children will help us to improve our playing if we let them.

Mechanistic play, especially isolated computer play, can work against children's creativity. Who is learning the most: the child with an expensive computer who can access the internet, or the child who 'invents' a computer with a cardboard box, wire and plasticine?

Adults in our drama groups need lots of reassurance, that they cannot get it 'wrong' and they might just have some fun. They are not being asked to be professional actors, but are using the well-tried skills of the actor to develop their communication and creativity. Let's take the following basic brainstorming and improvisation ideas and see what we can do with them.

'In the Picture' Activities

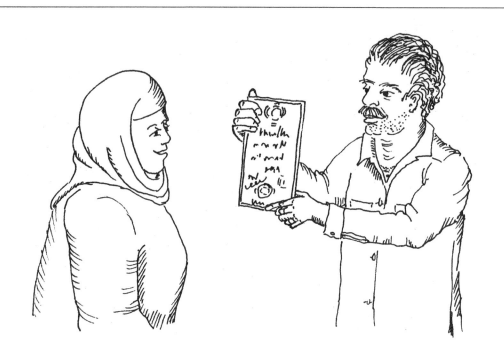

Photocopy Worksheet 8.1, which provides a copy of this picture, for each member of the group. (Don't forget to check the group's literacy levels first.) Every person then develops one of the following ideas.

- With a partner, explore together as many different ideas as possible of what the picture might be about – who are the two people? What is the document? What is their relationship? Where might they be? Is anyone speaking? Create a short interaction between them.

- With a partner, 'sculpt' the two people first and see whether you get ideas – that is, get in the body posture, create the expressions and see what happens. Did *doing* tell you more than *talking*?

'In the Picture' Activities
(continued)

- With a partner, imagine that this scene is taking place in the waiting area of a hospital. What is happening and what is on the paper? Improvise the scene either verbally or non-verbally.

- Focus on the document alone: expand your ideas to the limits of what it could be. Create your own document in detail by drawing or painting.

- Imagine that the picture is called *Surprise* – what might it be about?

- Imagine that the picture is called *Shock* – what might it be about?

- As a group, think of all the titles it could have.

- In small groups create a drama, with one person being the director and the other two being the characters in the picture. Improvise the storyline and let the director stop and start: for example, after a few moments of improvising, stop the action and suggest that both people are 20 years older or 10 years younger or are in the desert.

- In small groups think of the most ordinary storyline and improvise it. Then think of the most extraordinary and improvise that. Contrast the two interpretations and decide if one is more appropriate for this picture.

'In the Picture' Activities (continued)

All these exercises are helpful for encouraging creativity and improvisation skills. Use the chart on the following page to record people's progress in creativity and other qualities – or make a chart of your own. When recording 'Generosity' levels, observe whether people are generous with others with their ideas, or insist on clinging to their own. When recording 'Determination' levels, observe how well people stay with an idea, not giving up too easily.

Also encourage people to rate themselves, say, before the group starts and 10 sessions later. Take time to discuss all the words first to make sure that they are well understood. Include in the discussion the rationale for why these qualities are important in life.

Recording Chart
for Drama Groups

1–10 Scale Rating

Playfulness

1	2	3	4	5	6	7	8	9	10

Spontaneity

1	2	3	4	5	6	7	8	9	10

Creativity

1	2	3	4	5	6	7	8	9	10

Collaboration

1	2	3	4	5	6	7	8	9	10

Trust

1	2	3	4	5	6	7	8	9	10

Generosity

1	2	3	4	5	6	7	8	9	10

Determination

1	2	3	4	5	6	7	8	9	10

Innovation

1	2	3	4	5	6	7	8	9	10

This chart can be used with individuals and with groups.

Getting to Know the Characters' Activities

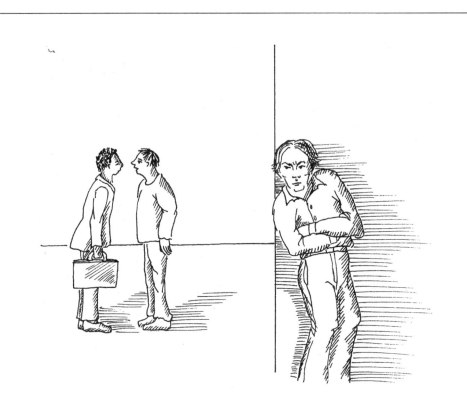

This picture is quite different from the previous one; like the previous picture, however, it is suggestive of many different situations. As in the last exercise, let everyone in the group have a copy of the picture (Worksheet 8.2) and then explore, through brainstorming and improvisation, the many possibilities.

- **Where** are these people? How did they get there? Is it a public space? Who else might be there?

- **When** is this interaction taking place? What time of day? What season of the year? What day of the week?

- **Why** are these people where they are? Have they arrived in this space by accident or is it planned? Why are they doing what they are doing?

Getting to Know the Characters' Activities (continued)

- **Who** are these people? Do they know each other? Are they related? How old are they? Are they men or women?

- **What** is the main focus of this story? Is there a 'subtext' to the scene (the scene 'underneath' the scene)? Are there other stories in the scene?

Tell the story from the point of view of each of the characters – in small groups; each group takes one character and tells their story. After this exploration see just how much more you know about the possibilities of this picture. Is there an interpretation that you feel is more authentic? More real? Too extreme? How well do you know these people?

Routledge
Taylor & Francis Group

Postcard Activities

Keep collections of different postcards for use in improvisation: the possibilities are endless. I have collections under the following headings:

- Contrasting landscapes – as many different ones as possible.

- Lots of trees, both real and imaginary.

- Family groups from as many cultures as possible.

- Doors and windows from all over the world.

- Keys to every type of door and box.

- Individual personalities – people who are: elderly, from different ethnic groups, different professions or in different contexts.

- Postcards with messages on the back – not your own of course! Some second-hand postcards have very interesting statements on them, making them ideal for improvisation.

- As many different animals as possible – including wild, domestic and farm animals. The animal pictures can be used to suggest different movement. How does this creature move? Which animals are antagonistic?

- Signposts, plaques and commemorative seals.

- People and landscapes that indicate a mood or a feeling.

Routledge
Taylor & Francis Group

Postcard Activities
(continued)

- All types of huts and houses – from palaces to squats.

- Clocks and watches in all shapes and sizes and of different ages.

- Pictures of pictures – famous paintings or portraits that evoke an event or a personality.

- If you have a random collection of cards, individuals or small groups can choose one card and use it for improvisation.

- If you have a themed session – for example, on 'Keys' – then let people choose a card 'blind'.

- Use the 'people cards' for improvisations to lead into role plays.

- The landscapes can be a context for improvisation of 'what happens in this place'.

- Houses can create a place for a story or the story may be about the house itself. Is it haunted? Who owns it? Who lives there?

These techniques can also be used for 'playing at home' – for adults to create dramatic play with children, to encourage confidence and narrative skills, both in the adults as well as the children.

Routledge Taylor & Francis Group

Group Improvisation Activities

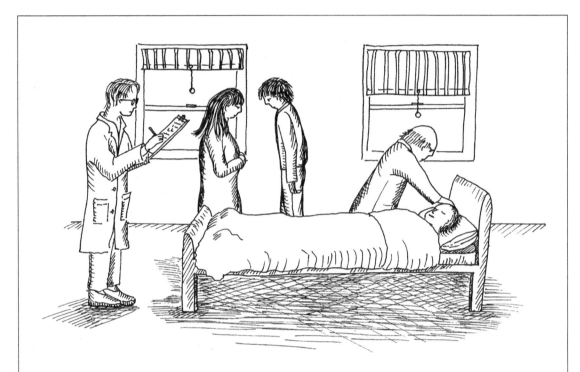

This picture can be improvised with a larger group of people, representing all five characters. Notice how we started with a scene with two people, then three, then five. It is important to start with pair work until people's confidence grows. Let everyone have a copy of the picture (Worksheet 8.3) and they will need time to think about the scene. It can then be explored in some of the following ways:

- Create some 'freeze frames' (sculpts) to show the beginning, middle and end of the story.

- Imagine this is a 'medical soap' (every television channel has several) – and improvise a typical scene in the style of the soap.

- Use the five 'W' questions we asked above: Where? When? Why? Who? What?

- How many stories are there in this picture?

Group Improvisation Activities (continued)

- Are the stories interlinked in other ways, or just in this picture?

- Think what view is outside the windows. Could the view alter the context inside the room?

- Play the scene as high comedy or slapstick.

- Think of different contexts for this scene, other than the medical.

- How does it change if one character is famous?

- Play the scene as if it is an opera.

- Play the scene as if it is on board ship.

- Make use of the picture to start an improvisation, and then use it to end an improvisation.

- Choose one character and create the scene as part of their life story.

- What else might be in the room – draw it to change the atmosphere.

Which of the improvisations seems to 'work' as an outcome of the picture? Create the opportunity to practise giving feedback about the drama so that it does not feel like personal criticism. This is a very important skill to develop in relation to drama work: we all know when it 'works' – and we do not have to settle for second best.

Routledge Taylor & Francis Group

The Fruits of Creative Improvisation

Having completed some of these activities, members of the groups will be more confident, not only at doing drama but also in appraising it: they will be more able to be self-critical as well as being able to critically appraise others. It will not happen immediately because we need to hone a lot of skills, as we have described in earlier chapters. We need to develop our voices as well as our bodies. We need to learn to play again, as well as taking risks with our ideas. Improvisation is about 'taking risks' in order to experiment and test whatever comes to mind.

Improvisation is also about developing our imagination, which is something that everyone has but in some people it is underdeveloped. People who have been traumatised can either be 'frozen' and too scared to allow their imagination to the fore, or may be at the other extreme, in which they are living in their imagination all the time! Drama and play work can help us leave these extremes and feel free to use our imagination when we choose, for what we want and where we need it.

Stream of Consciousness Writing

Stream of consciousness writing is similar to improvisation in drama: we freely allow the words or actions to be expressed without worrying about 'logic' or 'sequence'. We can practise 'free writing' about any of the scenes in these pictures. This process can be used in its own right or as a way of extending our ideas in the drama. People feel hesitant to be so free with their imaginations for several reasons. One is that they are easily anxious if sexual phrases come too readily to mind; another is that they are scared of being interpreted and 'analysed'. They are also scared of not 'getting it right', as we discussed earlier in this chapter.

Nonsense – or Not?

A good exercise to stimulate free writing is to have a heap of newspapers and some scissors. Cut out a pile of words from the newspapers and arrange them in a nonsense sequence or poem. Play with the words in every possible combination; turn them upside down so they are truly random phrases when you turn them over!

You will find that it is quite difficult to make nonsense: our brains always want the phrases to make sense and have logic of their own. Again we can develop our critical awareness and comment on the outcomes. Are they truly nonsense? It is far less threatening to discuss whether something is really nonsense, than to comment on whether it makes sense! Criticism from our schooldays still goes very deep with many people and they need time to move beyond these wounds. Plenty of affirmation and confidence building is the way to help to counterbalance negative feelings.

Perhaps it does us all good to remember our own negative experiences and how we managed to recover from them – if we have? Childhood is our most vulnerable time, and our early life is the most formative of all. Yet how often do we carry childhood scars into adulthood with no obvious means of remission? I cannot emphasise too much the importance of learning again to play as part of the repair process for adults.

'The Journey' Activities

The next picture in this chapter is called *The Journey* and can be used initially for creative writing and then improvisation. Use Worksheet 8.4 to work with ideas of the journey itself or of one person who is going on this journey. Use the 'W' questions to explore the picture and discuss whether the travellers have chosen to take this journey or had it imposed upon them. They seem mainly to be young people and children. Maybe they are out for the day? It has an air of a new journey to a promised land, but who is leading whom?

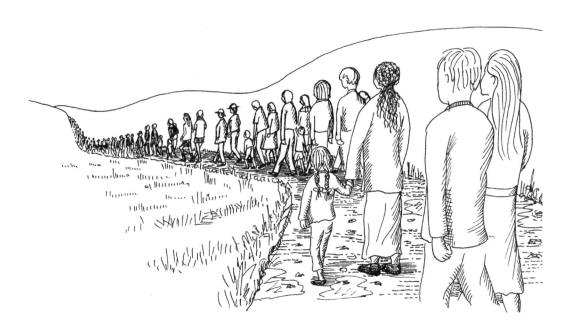

Worksheets 8.6 and 8.7 provide further 'journey' activities.

The Journey of Odysseus

The story of Odysseus' journey that took a total of twenty years, provides us with many dangers and crises to confront. There are many versions of this story (for example Walcott, 1993). Odysseus' son was a baby when he went away to the wars so now he is a young man. Will Odysseus recognise him when he eventually returns home to Ithaca? Odysseus sailed in a raft and was tempted to listen to the sirens' singing. They would bewitch sailors into leaving their boats, and then they would drown in the ocean depths.

Create an improvised story about his journey and all the things that might stop him returning to his native land. Give it a modern context too and think about what diverts us from getting on with want we really want to do.

If life is a journey, then what blocks and stops and diversions to we allow to get our way? This in itself can make a useful discussion, role play or improvisation.

Worksheet 8.1
In the Picture

Name _____ Date _____

_____

_____

_____

_____

_____

_____

_____

_____

You can continue your story on the back of this sheet.

Worksheet 8.2
Exploring the Characters

Name _____ Date _____

_____

_____

_____

_____

_____

_____

_____

You can continue your story on the back of this sheet.

Worksheet 8.3
Group Improvisation

Name _____ Date _____

_____

_____

_____

_____

_____

_____

_____

_____

_____

_____

You can continue your story on the back of this sheet.

Worksheet 8.4
The Mysterious Journey

Name _____ Date _____

Imagine that this picture is a scene at the docks, where
there is a ship getting ready for sailing on the tide.
Who are these people and what is everyone planning?
Where is the ship sailing to and for what purpose?
Use this as a basis for improvisation.

_____

_____

_____

_____

_____

_____

_____

_____

You can continue your story on the back of this sheet.

Worksheet 8.5
The Journey of Odysseus

Name _____ Date _____

The Voyage of Odysseus

Use the map of Odysseus' journey to create an improvisation of going across the seas on a strange journey: of meeting monsters and giants; distractions and temptations; ending with homecoming and welcome.

Write your ideas and use them to create a drama.

_____

_____

_____

_____

_____

_____

_____

_____

You can continue your story on the back of this sheet.

Routledge
Taylor & Francis Group

Worksheet 8.6
The Journey for the Treasure

Name _____ Date _____

Imagine that this document is a treasure map that has just been discovered. Improvise a journey to discover the treasure. It is for you to decide what type of treasure it is.

Make notes on you starting points for this journey before you develop your improvisation.
Compare your notes with others in your group and agree to combine some of the ideas.

_____

_____

_____

_____

_____

You can continue your story on the back of this sheet.

Routledge
Taylor & Francis Group

Worksheet 8.7
The Journey of a Lifetime

Name _____ Date _____

Draw a picture of a landscape postcard that you have been sent: one that took your fancy to such an extent that you can remember the detail.

Otherwise make up a postcard that you would like to receive.

Keep in your mind the idea that it is a landscape for a journey – a very special journey.

Use this landscape as a basis to create your own journey-map to a special place, *or* as a fantasy journey to somewhere you can go in your imagination.

Use as basis for improvisation.

Routledge Taylor & Francis Group

CHAPTER 9

Drama Techniques and Strategies

THIS CHAPTER IS ABOUT how we organise our drama workshops and the skills and structures that we need in order to realise the maximum potential of our groups and ourselves. The creative process is a two way process and taps into our own creativity as well as that of the people with whom we work. We cannot just 'do drama' out of a book as if it is a collection of recipes. This book is not meant to be a 'do it yourself' drama book. It provides ideas, themes, exercises and workshop plans, *but* it needs you, the reader, to bring it into being.

You are the guide or the energiser or facilitator who will assist your groups to breathe life into dramatic action. It is important to remember that an artistic process is at the core of the action and that your own artistry is important. I can almost hear the gasp of disbelief from some people because I use the word 'artistry'!

Overcoming Negativity

So many people come to my workshops and start with an apology, such as: 'I am just not creative', 'I can't act', 'I can't put one foot in front of the other so don't ask me to move' or 'Teachers always said I have no imagination'. The list is endless and so much of it stems from childhood experience.

Let's try another way into this self-deprecation and see if we can understand it. Sit quietly with a pen and paper and ponder the following questions before you answer them.

A. Creativity Negated

1 Can you recall a parent spending time playing with you: games, dramas, sports and so on?

_____

_____

2 How controlled were these activities? How much choice did you have in relation to 'free playing'?

_____

_____

3 What were your favourite playful and artistic activities when you were a small child? Were they lone activities or with other children/adults?

_____

_____

4 When you drew paintings at school was your work affirmed? Put on the wall? Praised by your parents?

_____

_____

5 Were you encouraged to attend classes, clubs or summer camps for dance, drama, painting, circus skills or other creative pursuits?

_____

_____

Routledge
Taylor & Francis Group

A. Creativity Negated
(continued)

6 How old were you when an adult first criticised your creativity: maybe essay writing, poetry, music, painting, dance, drama, sewing…?

_____

_____

7 Was your work ever compared unfavourably with a brother or sister or pupils at your school?

_____

_____

Find a way to share these negative experiences and see if you can 'move beyond them' – and I mean *move*. Dance your way into a more positive frame of mind or paint a new picture that can be your landscape or recognise that other people's negative perceptions belong to them and not to you.

Routledge
Taylor & Francis Group

B. Creativity Affirmed

1 Describe the joy of making a mess with mud, fingerpaints, or flour and water.

_____

_____

2 Did you have an invisible friend or a special toy that used to be a character in your playing?

_____

_____

3 Describe any 'special times' of play or story time with your parents.

_____

_____

4 Describe any favourite teachers who were inspiring and supportive of your creative work.

_____

_____

5 At what age did you start to write poems? Do you still have them?

_____

_____

B. Creativity Affirmed
(continued)

6 Did you create your own stories or enjoy those written by other people? Describe the stories that you really enjoy(ed).

_____

_____

7 How did you create play when you were a child? Were you the director or the actor or the playwright?

_____

_____

Is it possible to have enough of the positive experiences in section B to counteract the toxic effects of section A? Maybe there is only one positive thing in section B, but it may be strong enough to hold on to: creativity needs to be fed and stimulated. Unless we can develop our own artistry it will become dormant and will take much longer to revive. Rather like the old fashioned saying 'An apple a day keeps the doctor away', we could say to ourselves that 'Playing each day keeps madness at bay'!

If we really can recall no moment of light in our childhood creativity, we will have to work extra hard to turn that negativity around in our drama, movement and play.

Drama and play sessions need to be planned and it is important that we create a structure that relates to the aims and outcomes of our sessions. It is worthwhile to spend time writing down as much detail for ourselves as possible regarding the group and its activities.

The Drama Groups for Social and Recreational Purposes

If the main aim of the drama group is recreational, it is important for there to be a variety of activities. You and the group may be aiming to have some kind of presentation or performance at the end of a term or for the summer or for Christmas. You need to decide with the group on the basic ground rules: is it a fixed membership or can people come and go? What do the group want to get out of the sessions? Does it have mainly a social function or do people want to improve their skills? Do members know about the benefits of joining in a drama group?

Drama can have physical, psychological, spiritual and social benefits. These benefits can accrue from it just being a drama group, not a dramatherapy group. Creativity is one general outcome of such a group and that has a wide range of benefits. Drama can have a transforming effect on us as individuals as well as on the group as a whole. It helps us to grow, and to expand our perception of ourselves, and the world around us.

Drama and theatre are activities and artistic experiences that are 'worth doing' and the fact that they have existed for thousands of years shows their enduring value and tenacity. Although artistic experience is increasingly marginalised in our society, nevertheless it is still a vibrant and necessary resource for our continued well-being. Through drama and theatre we are able to create something unique even though we use a well-known text. It is our view of the text – something that we see from our perspective that makes it unique. We can only create this with the willing co-operation of others who will bring the text to life.

> The paradox is that we are creating something new from something old and that we feel a sense of familiarity that we knew it all the time!

We may want to start in a much smaller way: creating ideas for sculpts, for example. We have seen how we can sculpt the beginning, middle and end of the story. Just three movements can communicate the essence of a tale. We can use puppets or small figures to create the story that we then tell to others. We always need to remember to play.

It is important that these benefits are discussed with the group and may be photocopied as a handout or poster: people need as much information as possible, and need to be able to ask questions and maybe participate in a 'taster session'. It is not helpful to make the experience mysterious, otherwise people may well be suspicious and avoid participating: it might be a trick or make them look silly! Indeed it might.

Benefits of Participating in a Creative Drama Group

Physical Benefits

- Correct breathing improves circulation. It can also help to relieve asthma and chest complaints, sleep patterns, voice development and relaxation.

- Movement develops co-ordination, flexibility, circulation and balance.

- Brain development is influenced by creativity and playfulness.

Psychological Benefits

- Self-confidence and communication skills.

- Balance of emotions and thoughts.

- Empathy and understanding.

- Self-criticism and appraisal.

- Reworking of healthier attachments.

Spiritual Benefits

- Creativity allows us to go 'beyond ourselves'.

- Ritual drama can be a spiritual experience.

- Drama time is 'time out' from the everyday and mundane routine.

- Theatre has many roots in religious experience and texts.

Benefits of Participating in a Creative Drama Group (continued)

Social Benefits

- Drama is a collaborative activity.

- Participants have to communicate with each other and listen to one another.

- Very different people come together with a common aim and intention.

- There is a greater tolerance between people.

- Shared creativity gives a focus for talking and relationships.

Drama Groups for Therapeutic Purposes

Therapeutic Benefits of Participation in a Drama Group

Now that dramatherapy is a State Registered profession and a practice that is regulated by the Health Professions Council (HPC), people may not use the term 'dramatherapist' or 'dramatherapy' unless they have successfully completed a recognised training and are on the HPC register. This is the same for all the other arts therapies in the UK (music therapy, art therapy, dance-movement therapy). This is not the place to have a debate concerning these issues. The important thing is that it must not stop people facilitating drama and theatre workshops that can be described as 'therapeutic' rather than 'therapy'.

If we aim to provide a more therapeutic experience, then all of the above benefits still apply – what can be more therapeutic than to:

- Experience greater positive health?
- Feel more confidant?
- Feel 'uplifted'?
- Discover a commonality with others?

However, drama work may touch personal areas of an individual quite inadvertently: a story may remind someone of their own situation, a character may provide a frightening image, people may play the same role over and over again. These are situations that need to be carefully monitored – but kept within the drama workshop, rather than being turned into personal exploration. For example, the person who gets distressed by a scene can play an active role in that scene, have his or her feelings acknowledged and then move on, or be the director that scene.

> You are working with the exploration of the theme, the story or the role –
> rather than exploring the person's personal history.

If there is greater distress, then the person needs to be encouraged to take that to their counsellor or mentor. The distress is not ignored, it is acknowledged and then moved on. Remember that all of us can get tearful, angry or depressed when we witness plays, documentaries, soaps or ceremonies – that is part of the fabric of life. We are sentient beings, and many of us are helped by being able to express their feelings in the drama group, within the safety of the drama. However, we need to monitor the degrees of response and whether the person seems to have reasonable coping strengths. We can use Lahad's assessment for coping strengths, BASICP. (For a detailed description see *Creative Storytelling with Children at Risk*, Jennings, 2004d, pp 65–69.) We get very scared of emotional responses and the expression of feelings, when surely that is one of the aims of the work we are doing. We aim to provide people with the pathways to express a range of emotions through creative means.

Starters for Drama

Many people get anxious about the very beginning – what do I go into the room and say? How do I introduce it all? What if they won't do it? The simple answer is that the more you do it the easier it gets! However, I can appreciate the nervousness of the new beginner. I well remember when I used to write various options on my arm in case I got stuck! And that is the first idea to be clear about – the plan – and it is fine to write it down. For a detailed discussion on planning do look at *Creative Drama in Groupwork* (Jennings, 1986) as well as reflecting on the following ideas. It is fine to have your plan written down and with you when you run your group – it does not just miraculously come out of your mouth!

The most basic plan is: beginning – middle – end. The beginning is a warm-up of body and voice; the middle is the development of a story, theme or text; the end is the closure where we all return to ourselves again and prepare to meet the world outside.

- You need to choose a physical warm-up or drama game (there are many in the previous chapters) and it should have some bearing on the middle section. For example, you would not use a very vigorous warm-up when the theme of the story is a silent journey across the moors.
- There are plenty of ideas in this book for middle sections of a group session and they can be explored through many different techniques. Further ideas follow below.
- The closure is an important one to structure. People need time to wind down and emerge from their creative activities. People are encouraged to share what they thought and felt about the drama – not about themselves. Remember that we are trying to encourage a session that is not just 'me centred'. We can ask questions, such as, 'Was it convincing?', 'What else might we do with the scene?', 'Did we believe what we saw?' (that is, was it authentic?). The drama is the focus rather than the personal experience, although of course people may well say that they enjoyed it or felt angry or frustrated: it is important to have as much communication as possible.

Let's look now at some more ideas for developing that middle section – warm-ups are easy, and we need to move on from them.

There are more pictures which can be used for developing your drama sessions in the worksheets at the end of this chapter. You will soon get to the point where you can find your own pictures or cards or members of the group can bring in their own ideas.

'The Social Scene' Activities

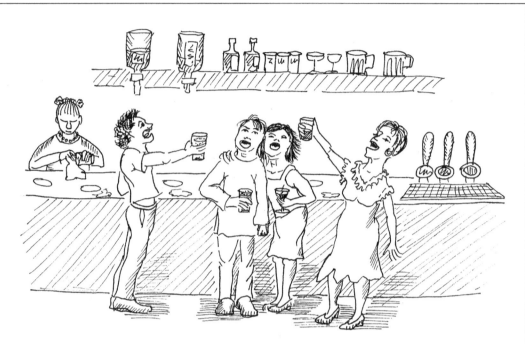

Photocopy Worksheet 9.1 and hand it out to the group. What is this scene about? Where is this happening? When is it taking place? Who are these people? Why have they gathered together? (Ask the five 'W' questions).

Is it a familiar scene? Does it take place on a regular basis? Is this place in the countryside, town or city? In which country does it take place?

Brainstorm the whole group or in small groups as much information as possible and then explore it actively through sculpting or through dramatisation. Continue further by seeing whether there is a fuller story to tell from the picture – is this the beginning or the end of a tale? Create a small play that includes this image – maybe it could be the start of a murder mystery or the middle of a successful robbery or the end of a birthday celebration. We always ask, 'What more is there?', 'What else can happen?'

> In drama and theatre we are extending everyone's possibilities so that life does not seem just a series of unhappy snapshots: things can grow and develop, they can go somewhere!

'Broken'
Activities

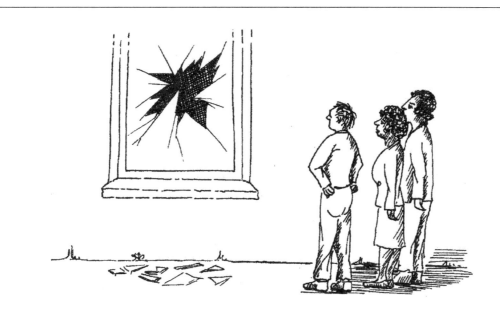

Now let's take a very different picture and explore our responses to it. In this picture there are fewer people and their expressions are very different! Study the picture and hand out photocopies of Worksheet 9.2; then discuss it. As with the previous picture, ask the five 'W' questions and then explore it in different ways.

- Discuss the ideas that this window may not belong to any of the people in the picture – they have simply discovered it.
- What if it is a window of an important or famous building?
- Is it just vandalism, or has someone gone inside? Perhaps a little difficult without getting cut! Or are there other discoveries?
- Initially, keep to what we can actually see in the picture to give the scene a focus.
- Then try to bring in other factors that are not visible, but may be associated.

Move on as soon as you can to explore this through drama rather than through talking – the range of possibilities you will find is more extensive and more creative.

> Try to keep the discussion to a minimum and explore in an active way
> through the drama: that is the philosophy, the theory and the practice. We
> learn more through drama and theatre than we can in any other way.

Routledge Taylor & Francis Group

P This page may be photocopied for instructional use only. *Creative Play & Drama with Adults at Risk* © Sue Jennings 2005

Things that Connect

Something that we all do as human beings is to make connections between things and this capacity is very useful in our drama work. Some people we work with have difficulty in making connections, others make very narrow connections. Both groups can be helped within the drama group to encourage this process of 'connectedness'. You can initially use pictures like the one below or you can carefully select a group of objects that will provide the framework for a story.

Having first done the physical and vocal warm-ups, a useful way into this process is to present the group with a box or tray of objects. Everyone chooses one object to improvise with. People can either choose an object or you can put them in a bag and they have to take one 'blind'. You can do the same with a broad selection of hats.

You can explore all different aspects of the objects and their relationship to each other. You can add on facts of your choice: for example, you might say that all these objects were found in a summer house in the grounds of a large house, or that they turned up at a car-boot sale. From this initial exploration, a story, a drama and then a piece of theatre will emerge. This early playing with ideas will enable a storyline and a situation of greater depth to be developed. You can choose which object to start with in the discussion; later, members of the group can choose, as they become more confident.

Again we return to the word 'playing'. It is really important that we keep this word to underpin everything we do in the drama group – we are encouraging people to be playful. It is through playfulness that they will experience the true joy of creation – and that is indeed a promotion of health! Playing and health is the first aim of the drama and theatre group.

'Connections'
Activities

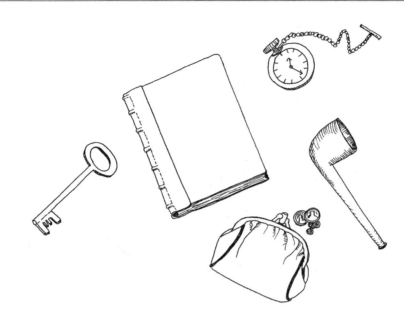

You are exploring with the group what the connection is between these objects – how is it they all belong to the same story. You may introduce them one or two at a time, otherwise people may think this is like a trick question where you have to quickly come up with an answer. When you have introduced all the objects, hand out copies of Worksheet 9.3.

- What sorts of people have a pipe and a watch-chain? How old are they? Where do they live? What time does the watch say? Is it significant? What is happening for this person who smokes the pipe and wears this watch?

- Does the key belong to the same person? Or do they find it? What is the significance of this key? Who does it belong to and why is it important?

- The purse may belong to someone else – who could it be? Does this second person know the person with the pipe? Why is some of the change out of the purse – was it dropped or taken?

- And the book: does that have a solution for us? It could be quite old – is it a diary? A valuable first edition? Maybe it has a connection with the key?

Routledge
Taylor & Francis Group

'The Story Behind the Objects' Activities

The following picture is very different but can be explored in exactly the same way. It may be that this set of objects all belong to the same person, and the group can explore who this character might be and what their story is. Other people can be a part of the story as it emerges.

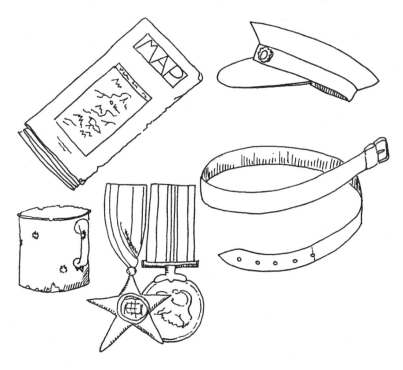

This picture (which appears on Worksheet 9.4) could also generate into variations on the activities. There might be a story about someone's life which could then be a play; there could be a story about a family and what happened; there could be a story about the medals and how they were won. There could also be a story about the breakdown of a relationship through death or separation. A husband and wife? A man and his grandfather? A father and his son?

The group could think about creating a documentary about this person's story – would it be a personal documentary or a war record?

Routledge
Taylor & Francis Group

Further Explorations

The possibilities are endless for this kind of exploration and you will find that stories will breed stories and will trigger other similar stories from things people have read or from their own families.

Worksheets 9.5–9.9 give plenty more ideas for what I call 'the drama of connections', which will turn into a very rich theatre experience. We become connected with other people in the drama group because we are all working together with a joint endeavour. Theatre itself is a huge exercise in social skills as we have to collaborate in order to get 'the show on the road' and on time!

It is not that drama is just a social activity where people can come together. It is the actual *doing of the drama* that enables greater social interaction to take place. We undergo profound changes in this process as I have earlier described, and it will continue to work. A colleague came to me only this week, saying:

> Sue, I am so pleased to have been able to join your drama group for a few weeks: it has completely turned my life around. I can now see something *so clearly*, that I can make a decision. It was all too jumbled up before!

This is a clear example of the impact of a drama group on someone's day-to-day life and decision-making.

> Drama and theatre help us to see the wood for the trees – through distancing we can come closer.

Worksheet 9.1
The Social Scene

Name _____ Date _____

_____

_____

_____

_____

_____

_____

_____

_____

_____

_____

_____

You can continue your story on the back of this sheet.

Worksheet 9.2
Broken

Name _____ Date _____

_____

_____

_____

_____

_____

_____

_____

_____

_____

You can continue your story on the back of this sheet.

Routledge
Taylor & Francis Group

P This page may be photocopied for instructional use only. *Creative Play & Drama with Adults at Risk* © Sue Jennings 2005

Worksheet 9.3
Connections

Name _____ Date _____

_____

_____

_____

_____

_____

_____

_____

_____

You can continue your story on the back of this sheet.

Worksheet 9.4
The Story Behind the Objects

Name _____ Date _____

_____

_____

_____

_____

_____

_____

You can continue your story on the back of this sheet.

Routledge
Taylor & Francis Group

P

Worksheet 9.5
Characters and Scenes

Name _____ Date _____

Who is this person? Can he hear and is he talking to someone who cannot hear? Or is he trying to tell somebody something? What do you think is being said? Is it urgent? Create this character and think about what scene they could be in.

To get some experience of what it is like to be without hearing, put earplugs in and watch everyone else talking. Another way is for everyone else to mouth what they are saying so there is no sound – or watch television with the sound turned down.

_____

_____

_____

_____

You can continue your story on the back of this sheet.

Routledge
Taylor & Francis Group
P

Worksheet 9.6
More Characters and Scenes

Name _____   Date _____

This is a girl, but who is she? Is she dressed up as a fairy? Is it her dancing class? Is she a fairy in a story and this is an illustration? Explore as many ideas as you can and then write her story. Either direct the story as a play with your group or enact the character yourself, with others.

_____

_____

_____

_____

_____

_____

You can continue your story on the back of this sheet.

Routledge
Taylor & Francis Group

Worksheet 9.7
Making Connections

Name _____ Date _____

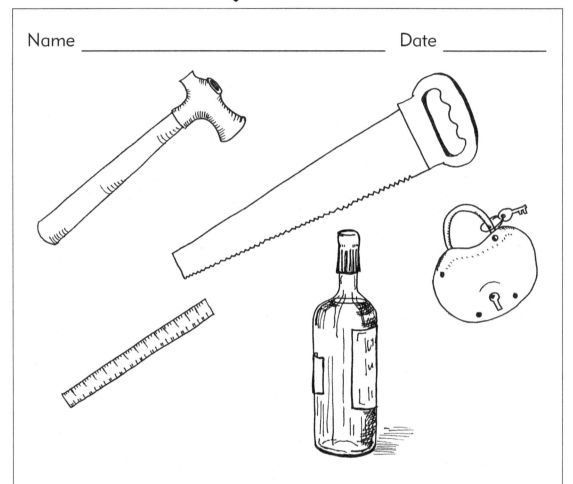

You can have many different connections to the objects in this picture. Perhaps the first question to ask is what is in the bottle? Play with the ideas of several different substances and see what a difference this might make to the story. Is there a relationship between the padlock and the bottle? Or the padlock and the tools? Or is the padlock the significant object that changes the story?

See which story fits with your view and then test it out with others and see if they have similar or very different ideas. Choose one version to turn into a play.
This exercise can also be explored with two people or in a small group.

Worksheet 9.8
Making More Connections

Name _____ Date _____

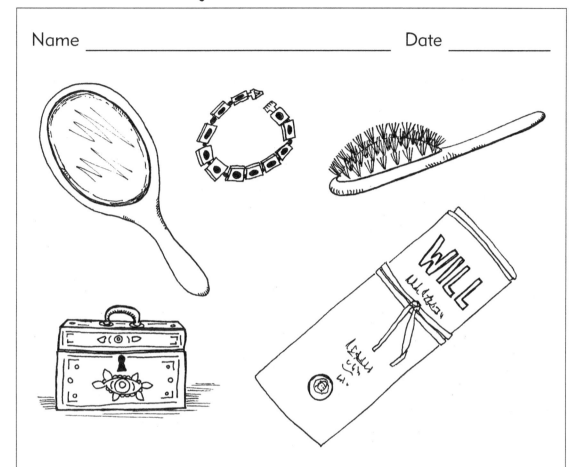

Where do you think these objects were found? Maybe under someone's bed? At the back of a wardrobe? At a murder scene? Three, perhaps four things could be associated with a dressing table, so whose room might these things have belonged to? Has the necklace come out of the box? Does the will belong to the person who owns the other objects, or does it belong to someone else? Is that a necklace, and if so what is it made of?

Create a mystery story that can be enacted with your group and try to create an unexpected ending.

Routledge
Taylor & Francis Group

Worksheet 9.9
The Drama of Connections

Name _____ Date _____

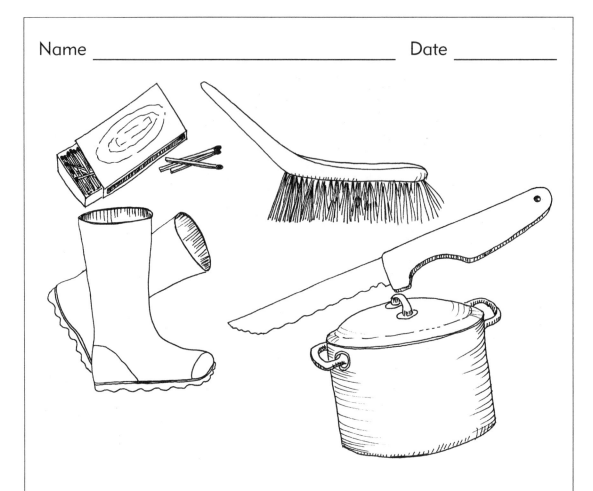

Try agreeing where the place is for all these objects before you decide on their owner. For example, they could all be in the shed in someone's garden or yard, or they could be tagged evidence to produce in a courtroom. Then decide on their connections – they are not things that we would necessarily put together. Where do the matches fit into it? What is the metal vessel? What are the boots made of? Do they belong to a man or a woman?

Make group decisions about the storyline and then turn it into a piece of drama with several characters.

Routledge
Taylor & Francis Group

CHAPTER 10

Play, Theatre and Performance

I N THIS CHAPTER I EMPHASISE the importance of not only drama but also theatre in our work with people 'at risk'. Many people have difficulty in naming theatre as a healing medium and an agency of change. I know from my own personal experience that theatre can bring about major life changes.

The Experience of Theatre

Theatre is multi-dimensional: it involves the biological and the spiritual, the social and the ritualistic, the artistic and the aesthetic. It is about how we think as well as how we feel; it influences us as individuals as well as groups; it gives us security in the known as well as allowing us to experience the unknown. Theatre is a part of our culture and one that is rapidly taking on new forms, especially through the increase of technology.

Theatre is a social art: it needs others there to witness it; audience and actors develop a rapport that moves the play forward when it is working well. Theatre is a contained art form, it is encapsulated both in time and space, and the dramatic structure provides a beginning, middle and end. At the end of a play we can walk away; we may be moved, bored, enraged or excited, but we are disengaging from the process. The moment the actors appear out of character (though still in costume) to take their bow, we start to disengage.

Theatre always affects us in some way, even if we are not enjoying the play. It will make an impact on us in a way that other media cannot. Cinema and television have not replaced theatre: it is a question of 'both/and' rather than 'either/or'. Those that see it as a dominantly middle-class activity are marginalising live theatre, which has always evolved as society evolves. Live theatre may be for entertainment or social or political education. It may challenge the *status quo* or it may transform our experience through the sheer power of the aesthetic experience. It may indeed fulfil all of these aims within the same performance.

We need to remember that an experience in live theatre is always unique: the performance will change with every audience that is present, because theatre is born in that relationship between actors and audience. There is a meeting between the performers and the audience.

Theatre and Aesthetics

We go to the theatre and an aesthetic experience makes us come away feeling and thinking in new ways: it may well be 'art-for-art's sake', but we have shared this experience with a large or small group of other audience members. We are witnesses of a process that is being created in front of us and that may 'work' on one night but not on another. We can feel 'transported', taken to another place, and the themes and metaphors make some kind of impact. We are sitting more or less still in the theatre yet the words 'transport' and 'metaphor' are all about movement: the spirit and the psyche are shifting and we shall never be quite the same again.

The theatre encapsulates a total story or slice of life in a way that it can be managed within, say, the 'two hours traffic, of our stage' (Shakespeare, *Romeo and Juliet* 1, Prologue).

As Wilshire says:

Life itself is too large and strung out to be taken in as a whole by the mind.
(Wilshire, 1982)

Theatre with People with Special Needs

If we create theatre with people who have special needs, how does it actually work in practice? Is it theatre in its own right or is it dramatherapy?

Shakespeare's *A Midsummer Night's Dream* is a play that I have used with many groups of people, including offender patients at Broadmoor Hospital (Jennings, McGinley and Orr, 1997) and prison projects, children with learning disabilities and street children in India, and for personal development for professional groups. This play is very dark: it starts with a dysfunctional and violent family and culminates in key people running away to the forest. The forest contains all the fairy people, creatures from the spirit world, who have also become violent and threatening. A group of workmen have arrived in the forest to rehearse their play, which they want to perform at the Duke's wedding (an example of 'the play with the play'). In Chapter 3 I have discussed how this scene may be used in parallel with the Midas story (see pages 42–44).

Fresh Insights

There are dark forces in the forest, there is gratuitous violence and cruel game playing; love is betrayed and people's worlds turned upside down. Chaos ensues. Finally, after the fairy spirit world is at peace, all the humans come out of the forest, changed and reconciled, having seen and experienced things in a new way. Although the human world has returned to some predictability; there are fresh insights, new relationships and celebrations. Yet it is Bottom the weaver who says, 'I have had a most rare vision'. The insight has come from the workman, and he too has 'a midsummer night's dream'!

The last word typically comes from the trickster character in the play, Puck or Robin Goodfellow, who has created mayhem and chaos, but at the very end gives us a way of dealing with our experience. It is Puck who has created the chaos and then returns everything to order:

If we shadows have offended,
Think but this and all is mended:
That you have but slumbered here
While these visions did appear,
And this weak and idle theme,
No more yielding but a dream,
Gentles do not reprehend.
If you pardon, we will mend.
And as I am an honest puck,
If we have unearned luck
Now to 'scape the serpent's tongue,
We will make amends ere long,
Else the puck a liar call.
So, good night unto you all.
Give me your hands, if we be friends,
And Robin shall restore amends.
(Shakespeare, *A Midsummer Night's Dream* 5. i. 412–426)

Puck is telling us that if the play offends us then we should imagine that we have been sleeping and dreaming (the play is called 'The Dream'). Use the above as a poem in your group (Worksheet 10.1). Everyone can read it out together, or everyone can read it out together and look at someone to whom they are speaking the poem.

In this play there are some compromises and some rewards, but the end of the play not only allows the characters back into their ordinary worlds after the mysterious and magical forest; it also allows us, the audience, to remember that we are the audience. This process starts even earlier when Puck says to us:

Now the hungry lion roars,
And the wolf behowls the moon,
Whilst the heavy ploughman snores,
All with weary task foredone.
Now the wasted brands do glow
Whilst the screech-owl, screeching loud,
Puts the wretch that lies in woe
In remembrance of a shroud.
Now it is the time of night
That the graves, all gaping wide,
Everyone lets forth his sprite
In the churchway paths to glide;
And we fairies that do run
By the triple Hecate's team
From the presence of the sun,
Following darkness like a dream
Now are frolic. Not a mouse
Shall disturb this hallowed house.
I am sent with broom before
To sweep the dust behind the door.
(Shakespeare, *A Midsummer Night's Dream*, 5. i. 364–384)

This speech is a poem in itself and can be read and reflected on in its own right. It can be decorated or painted and the various metaphors explored as in Worksheet 10.2.

However, within the context of the story, this speech begins the closure process of the play. Puck describes to us the coming of night and the playfulness of the fairies. But then he addresses the audience directly: 'Not a mouse/Shall disturb this hallowed house'. The house is the theatre (we speak of a 'full house'), and Puck is reassuring members of the audience that they will not be 'disturbed'. He is assisting the 'de-roling' process.

This closure is complete in Puck's second speech within the same scene, when he again addresses the audience directly, 'Give me your hands if we be friends'. This is the penultimate line of the play. He asks us to applaud the show and the players, and he will make good any shortcomings for the next performance.

This is the only play by Shakespeare where the closure is made so explicit and it is important to note that this is a play that has taken us into magical worlds. Shakespeare himself is bringing us back to 'everyday reality' after our journey through the forest. This play has 'dark materials', not only in the magical worlds but also in the families themselves. Every group that I have worked with has asked the question, 'Where are the mothers of the two girls, Hermia and Helena?' Their fathers are both present – one in person and one by name. One of the groups wanted to start their improvisation by exploring the family of Hermia: the absent mother and the anger of her father.

Through the 'distancing' of theatre we can see how this play allows us both to explore families who are in chaos and embark on a journey through the fairy world, without breaking down our own personal self. The distancing allows us to explore and to develop new experiences within the safety of the text and story.

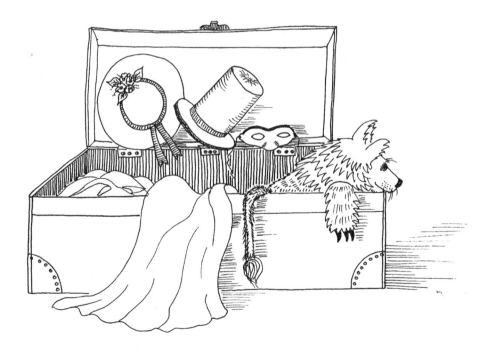

We can use the play as a whole and slowly build up the story or we can take specific scenes or certain speeches, like the two quoted above. If you are anxious or not engaged with the idea of playing Shakespeare, go and see a good production or look at one of the recent films, and see what happens!

All we need for playmaking is a box of clothes, props and perhaps some masks. These will all fire our imagination and the journey can start.

Endpiece

Try this idea for yourself and then see if you can try it with your groups. The following scene comes from Shakespeare's *Romeo and Juliet*.

Juliet's father, who is from the Capulet family, is having a big party and has invited all his friends and family. He is hoping that soon they will announce Juliet's engagement to Paris. It is a massive masked ball, with plenty of good food and wine and everyone is wearing ball gowns or velvet suits.

Romeo, who is a Montague, and his two friends Mercutio and Benvolio, decide to go the party of this rival family, wearing their masks and looking for mischief. They slip into the party and, since everyone is wearing masks, they are hardly noticed.

Juliet's father and mother and her uncle are at the party, and so is her nanny; there is also her cousin Tybalt who has a very fiery temper. Romeo is a romantic, Mercutio is a tease and a joker, and Benvolio tries to keep the peace.

Mask Activity

Decide on a character and make yourself a mask that you will wear to the ball. Take your time and decorate it how you will. Imagine that you are going to the ball and the people that you will meet. What liaisons are going on once the wine begins to flow? We know that Juliet and Romeo meet, and we also know that Tybalt notices Romeo. Think about this particular scene of the play from the point of view of your particular character, and write down your ideas and observations. Whose side are you on?

Now everyone can create the scene of the ball, wearing their finest clothes and making very formal introductions. You can then create a circle dance and with very simple side steps, remembering that you are wearing a very heavy costume. Discuss how you feel in these costumes, in the formal atmosphere, knowing that some kind of plot is brewing! Create your own intrigue and use it as the basis for an improvisation or enactment.

New Journey

Now read through the following speech, which is usually spoken by a chorus as a Prologue to the play (this can be photocopied from Worksheet 10.3):

Two households both alike in dignity,
(in fair Verona where we lay our scene)
From ancient grudge, break to new mutiny,
Where civil blood makes civil hands unclean:
From forth the fatal loins of these two foes,
A pair of star-cross'd lovers, take their life:
Whose misadventur'd piteous overthrows,
Doth with their death bury their parents' strife.
The fearful passage of their death-mark'd love,
And the continuance of their parents' rage:
Which but their children's end nought could remove:
Is now the two hours traffic of our Stage.
The which if you with patient ears attend
What here shall miss, our toil shall strive to mend.
(Shakespeare, *Romeo and Juliet*, Prologue)

What does it feel like to read a prologue at the end of the book? I hope it means that you are about to begin a new journey of play, drama and theatre: both for yourself and for your groups.

Worksheet 10.1
Puck's Promises

Name _____ Date _____

Read this speech out together as a group or suggest that one person can read it and the other can move to the rhythm. You can also decorate your poem.

If we shadows have offended,

Think but this and all is mended:

That you have but slumbered here

While these visions did appear,

And this weak and idle theme,

No more yielding but a dream,

Gentles do not reprehend.

If you pardon, we will mend.

And as I am an honest puck,

If we have unearned luck

Now to 'scape the serpent's tongue,

We will make amends ere long,

Else the puck a liar call.

So, good night unto you all.

Give me your hands, if we be friends,

And Robin shall restore amends.

(Shakespeare, *A Midsummer Night's Dream* 5. i. 412–426)

Worksheet 10.2
Night-time

Name _____ Date _____

What picture could illustrate this scene that Puck is describing?

Now the hungry lion roars,
And the wolf behowls the moon,
Whilst the heavy ploughman snores,
All with weary task foredone.

Now the wasted brands do glow
Whilst the screech-owl, screeching loud,
Puts the wretch that lies in woe
In remembrance of a shroud.
Now it is the time of night
That the graves, all gaping wide,
Everyone lets forth his sprite
In the churchway paths to glide;

And we fairies that do run
By the triple Hecate's team
From the presence of the sun,
Following darkness like a dream
Now are frolic. Not a mouse
Shall disturb this hallowed house.
I am sent with broom before
To sweep the dust behind the door.

(Shakespeare, *A Midsummer Night's Dream*, 5. i. 364–384)

Routledge Taylor & Francis Group P This page may be photocopied for instructional use only. *Creative Play & Drama with Adults at Risk* © Sue Jennings 2005

Worksheet 10.3
The Beginning of the End

Name _____ Date _____

Use this speech as a model of how to 'set the scene' at the beginning of the play.

A chorus can be one person or a group; experiment with both and see which you would choose for your play.

Perform the speech with different people each line.

Do remember the rhythm of the words and the number of beats each line.

Two households both alike in dignity,

(in fair Verona where we lay our scene)

From ancient grudge, break to new mutiny,

Where civil blood makes civil hands unclean:

From forth the fatal loins of these two foes,

A pair of star-cross'd lovers, take their life:

Whose misadventur'd piteous overthrows,

Doth with their death bury their parents' strife.

The fearful passage of their death-mark'd love,

And the continuance of their parents' rage:

Which but their children's end nought could remove:

Is now the two hours traffic of our Stage.

The which if you with patient ears attend

What here shall miss, our toil shall strive to mend.

(Shakespeare, *Romeo and Juliet*, Prologue)

CHAPTER 11

Useful Addresses

THE FOLLOWING IS A selective list of organisations which run short courses in drama, dramatherapy and action work. For information regarding play and play therapy please look at *Creative Storytelling with Children at Risk* (Jennings, 2004d).

Actionwork *(Regional, International)*
PO Box 433
Weston Super Mare
Somerset
BS24 0WY
+44 (0) 1934 815163
www.actionwork.com

Family Futures Consortium
(London and National)
35 Britannia Road
Islington
London
N1 8QH
+44 (0) 207 354 4161
www.familyfutures.co.uk

Institute for Arts and Therapy in Education
2–18 Britannia Row
Islington
London
N1 8PA
+44 (0) 207 704 2534
www.artspyschotherapy.org

Millbrook House
(formerly St Loye's School of Health Studies)
School of Health Professions
Facultyof Health and Social Work
University of Plymouth
Millbrook Lane
Exeter
Devon
EX2 6ES
+44 (0) 1392 219774
www2.plymouth.ac.uk/millbrook/

The Northern Trust for Dramatherapy
The Registrar Manchester
University Course
41 Netheroyd Hill Road
Fixby
Huddersfield
HD2 2LS
+44 (0) 1484 428427

Rowan Studio
(Somerset, National and International)
63A Westmoreland Terrace
London
SW1V 4AH
+44 (0) 20 7592 9514

Sesame, The Central School of Speech and Drama
Embassy Theatre
Eton Avenue
London
NW3 3HY

+44 (0) 207 722 8183
www.cssd.ac.uk

SkillsActive (formerly SPIRITO)
(Head Office)
Castlewood House
77–91 New Oxford Street
London
WC1A 1PX

+44 (0) 207 632 2000
www.skillsactive.com

Society for Storytelling
PO Box 2344
Reading
RG6 7PG

+44 (0) 1752 569 244
sfs@fairbruk.demon.co.uk
www.sfs.org.uk

Workshops, newsletter, very active email news.

University of Derby
Student Office
Western Road
Mickleover
Derby
DE3 5GX

+44 (0) 1332 592040
www.derby.ac.uk

University of Roehampton
(Surrey)
Southlands College
80 Roehampton Lane
London
SW15 5SL

+44 (0) 208 392 3807
www.roehampton.co.uk

CHAPTER 12
Bibliography
References and Further Reading

Axline V, 1964, *Dibs in Search of Self,* Penguin, London.

Bannister A & Huntington A, 2002, *Communicating with Children and Adolescents: Action for Change,* Jessica Kingsley, London.

Barker, 1977, *Theatre Games,* Methuen Drama, London.

Berg O, 1998, 'Personal Communication', OEMP Conference, Copenhagen, Denmark.

Boal A, 1992, *Games for Actors and Non-Actors,* Routledge, London.

Brooking-Payne K, 1996, *Games Children Play,* Hawthorn Press, Stroud.

Campbell J, 1959/1969/2000, *Primitive Mythology,* Souvenir Press, London.

Campbell J, 1962, *Oriental Mythology,* Souvenir Press, London.

Campbell J, 1968/2001, *Creative Mythology,* Souvenir Press, London.

Campbell J, 1964, *Occidental Mythology,* Souvenir Press, London.

Carson R, 1965, *Silent Spring,* Penguin, Harmondsworth.

Casson J, 2001, Book Review: *The Actors are Come Hither,* by Walton P, *The Prompt,* Winter.

Casson J, 2004, *Drama, Psychotherapy and Psychosis,* Brunner-Routledge, Hove and New York.

Cattanach A, Chesner A, Jennings S, Mitchell S & Meldrum B, 1994, *The Handbook of Dramatherapy,* Routledge, London.

Chesner A, 1994, *Drama for People with Learning Disabilities,* Speechmark, Bicester.

Courtney R, 1981, 1990, *Re-Play,* Oise Press, Toronto.

Courtney R & Schattner G, 1982a, *Drama in Therapy: Volume 1 Children,* Drama Book Specialists, New York.

Courtney R & Schattner G, 1982b, *Drama in Therapy: Volume 2 Adults,* Drama Book Specialists, New York.

Cox M, 1992, *Shakespeare Comes to Broadmoor,* Jessica Kingsley, London.

Cozolino L, 2002, *The Neuroscience of Psychotherapy,* WW Norton, New York.

Duggan M & Grainger R, 1997, *Imagination, Identification and Catharsis,* Jessica Kingsley, London.

Edgar D, 1978, *Mary Barnes,* Methuen, London.

Elsie R (trans), 2001, *Albanian Folktales and Legends,* Dukagjini Printing, Kosovo.

Friedlander G, 2001, *Jewish Fairy Tales,* Dover Publications, New York.

Garland C, 2001, an interview in *Woman and Home,* April.

Gerhardt S, 2004, *Why Love Matters: how affection shapes a baby's brain,* Brunner-Routledge, London.

Gersie A, 1991, *Storymaking in Bereavement,* Jessica Kingsley, London.

Gersie A, 1992, *Earth Tales,* Green Press, London.

Gersie A, 2002, 'The Nine Part Story Structure', *The Prompt,* Summer.

Gersie A & King N, 1990, *Theories of Childhood,* Redleaf Press, Minnesota.

Grainger R, 1995, *The Glass of Heaven: The Faith of the Dramatherapist,* Jessica Kingsley, London.

Hansen T, 1991, *Seven for a Secret: Healing the wounds of sexual abuse in childhood,* SPCK, London.

Hathaway N, 2002, *The Friendly Guide to Mythology,* Penguin, London.

Hickson A, 1995, *Creative Action Methods in Groupwork,* Speechmark, Bicester.

Hickson A, 1997, *The Groupwork Manual,* Speechmark, Bicester.

Hickson A, 2002, *Silent Scream,* Video, Actionwork, Bleadon.

Hillman, J, 1983, *Healing Fiction,* Station Publications, New York.

Holaday D, Chin Woon Ping & Teoh Boon Seong, 2003, *Bes Hyang Dney and other Jah Hut Stories,* Center for Orang Asli Concerns, Malaysia.

Jennings S, 1973/2004, *Remedial Drama,* A&C Black/Play Therapy Press.

Jennings S (ed), 1975, *Creative Therapy,* Pitman/Kemble Press, Banbury.

Jennings S, 1979, 'Ritual and the Learning Process', *Journal of Dramatherapy,* 13.4.

Jennings S, 1986, *Creative Drama in Groupwork,* Speechmark, Bicester.

Jennings S (ed), 1987, *Dramatherapy Theory and Practice,* Vol 1, 2, 3, Routledge, London.

Jennings S, 1990, *Dramatherapy with Families, Groups and Individuals,* Jessica Kingsley, London.

Jennings S, 1991, 'Legitimate Grieving? Working with Infertility', Papadata D & Papadatos C (eds), *Children and Death,* Hemisphere Publishing Corporation, New York.

Jennings S (ed), 1992, *Dramatherapy Theory and Practice,* Vol 2, Routledge, London.

Jennings S & Minde A, 1993, *Art Therapy and Dramatherapy: Masks of the Soul,* Jessica Kingsley, London

Jennings S, 1993/2006, *Playtherapy with Children: a practitioner's guide,* Blackwell/Play Therapy Press, Fairwarp.

Jennings S (ed), 1995a, *Dramatherapy with Children and Adolescents,* Routledge, London.

Jennings S, 1995b, *Theatre, Ritual and Transformation,* Routledge, London

Jennings S, 1997, *Dramatherapy Theory and Practice,* Vol 3, Routledge, London.

Jennings S, McGinley J, Orr M, 1997, 'Dramatherapy and Offender Patients', *Dramatherapy Theory and Practice,* Vol 3, Routledge, London.

Jennings S, 1998, *Introduction to Dramatherapy: Ariadne's Ball of Thread,* Jessica Kingsley, London.

Jennings S, 1999, *Introduction to Developmental Playtherapy: Playing for Health,* Jessica Kingsley, London.

Jennings S, 2000a, *Brigid: Fertility, Creativity and Healing,* Rowan Studio, Glastonbury.

Jennings S, 2000b, 'Theatre at the Borders: Conflict resolution and social change', Bernardi C, Gragone M & Schinina G (eds), *War Theatres and Actions for Peace,* Eurisis Edizione, Milan.

Jennings S, 2001a, *Inanna: Journey into Darkness and Light,* Rowan Studio, Glastonbury.

Jennings S, 2001b, *Embodiment-Projection-Role,* training video, Actionwork, Bleadon.

Jennings S, 2001c, 'Healing Theatre', *Journal of Avalon,* Winter.

Jennings S, 2002, 'Play and the Brain: Developmental Shakespeare' presented at the Oslo Symposium 'Arts and the Brain'.

Jennings S, 2003a, 'EPR – A Model for Dramatic Play', *Play Words,* April/May.

Jennings S, 2003b, 'Playlore: The Roots of Humanity', *Play for Life,* Autumn.

Jennings S, 2003c, 'Playlore: The Sensory Foundation', *The Prompt,* Winter, 2003/2004.

Jennings S, 2004a, 'Playtherapy in Romania', *Play Words,* February/March.

Jennings S, 2004b, 'Social Play and Inclusion', *Play Words,* May/June.

Jennings S, 2004c, *Embodiment – Projection – Role with Children,* training video, Actionwork, Bleadon.

Jennings S, 2004d, *Creative Storytelling with Children at Risk,* Speechmark, Bicester.

Jennings S, 2004e, 'It's Hard to Make Roots', Dramatherapy, Playtherapy and Creative Theatre, Schinina G (ed), *Psychosocial Support to Groups of Victims of Human Trafficking,* Volume 4, February, IOM, Geneva.

Jennings S, 2004f, 'Stages of Surprise' (in English and German), Eberhart H & Killias H (eds), *Uberraschung als Anstoss zu Wandlungsprozessen,* Egis Verlag, Zurich.

Jennings S, 2005a, *Creative Storytelling with Adults at Risk,* Speechmark, Bicester.

Jennings S, 2005b, *The Playing Brain,* paper presented to conference 'Essential Play', University of Chichester.

Jennings S, 2005c, *Goddesses: Ancient Wisdom in Times of Change,* Hay House, London and San Francisco.

Jennings S, 2005d, *Creative Journeys: Meditation Stories for Children,* CD, Fasterbytes, Somerset.

Jennings S, 2005e, *Mrs Apple tells Stories,* CD, Fasterbytes, Somerset.

Jennings S & Hickson A, 2002, 'Pause for Thought: Action or Stillness with Young People', *Communicating with Children and Adolescents,* Bannister A & Huntingdon A (eds), Jessica Kingsley, London.

Johnstone K, 1981/1989, *Impro: Improvisation and the Theatre,* Methuen Drama, London.

Jung C, *Collected Works 1953–1979,* University Press, Princeton.

Jung C (trans), 1963, *Memories, Dreams and Reflections,* Pantheon, New York.

Lahad M, 1992, 'Story-making and assessment method for coping with stress', in *Dramatherapy: Theory and Practice,* Vol 2, Jennings S (ed), Tavistock/Routledge, London.

Lahad M, 2000, *Creative Supervision,* Jessica Kingsley, London.

Landy R, 1993, *Persona and Performance: The Meaning of Role in Drama, Therapy and Everyday Life,* Jessica Kingsley, London.

Meade EH, 1995, *Tell It by Heart: Women and the Healing Power of Story,* Open Court Publishing, Chicago.

Mellon N, 2000, *Storytelling with Children,* Hawthorn Press, Stroud.

Meyer R, 2001, *The Wisdom of Fairy Tales,* Floris Books, Edinburgh.

Moreno, JL, 1934, *Psychodrama,* Vol 1, Beacon House Press, New York.

Muten B (ed), 1999, *Her Words,* Shambhala, Boston and London.

Nesbit E, 1995, *The Railway Children,* Penguin Books, London.

Newham P, 1999, *The Healing Voice,* Vega, London.

O'Neill C, Casterton P & Headlam C (eds), 1998, *The Kingfisher Book of Mythology: Gods, Goddesses and Heroes from around the World,* Kingfisher, London.

Pitruzella A, 2004, *Introduction to Dramatherapy: Person and Threshhold,* Routlege, London.

Russell Davis D, 1992, *Scenes of Madness: A Psychiatrist at the Theatre,* Routledge, London.

Schechner R, 1985, *Between Theatre and Anthropology,* Philadelphia University Press, Philadelphia.

Schechner R, 1991, 'Magnitudes of Performance', *By Means of Performance,* New York, Cambridge University Press.

Schinina G, 2004, 'In Between … Working with Survivors of Trafficking in Transit Situations', Schinina G (ed), *Psychosocial Support to Groups of Victims of Human Trafficking,* Volume 4, February, IOM Geneva.

Shakespeare W, *Hamlet, A Midsummer Night's Dream, The Winter's Tale, As You Like It,* Penguin, London.

Simpson J, 1998, *Touching the Void,* Vintage, London.

Slade P, 1954, *Child Drama,* Hodder & Stoughton, London.

Spolin V, 1963, *Improvisation for the New Theater,* North Western University Press, Everston.

Stanislavski C, 1961, *Creating a Role,* Methuen, London.

Stanislavski C, 1981, *Building a Character,* Methuen, London.

Steinberg D, 2002, Personal Communication.

Sunderland M, 2000, *Using Story Telling as a Therapeutic Tool with Children,* Speechmark, Bicester.

Tambiah SJ, 1985, *Culture, Thought and Social Action,* Harvard University Press, MA.

Taylor P, 2003, *Applied Theatre,* Heinemann, London and Portsmouth NH.

Thompson J (ed), 1994, *Prison Theatre: Perspective and Practices,* Jessica Kingsley, London.

Turner V, 1982, 'From Ritual to Theatre', *New York Performing Arts Journal.*

Vygotsky LS, 1978, *Mind in Society,* Cole M (ed), Harvard University Press, Cambridge MA.

Walcott D, 1993, *The Odyssey,* Faber and Faber, London and Boston.

Walton P, 1998, *The Actors are Come Hither,* Biography of Elsie Green, Walton Press, Leatherhead.

Watts P, 1992, *Therapy in Drama in Dramatherapy, Theory and Practice 2,* Jennings S (ed), Routledge, London.

Wilshire B, 1982, *Role Playing and Identity: The Limits of Theatre as Metaphor,* Indiana University Press, Bloomington.

Winnicott D, 1974, *Playing and Reality,* Pelican, London.

97808638855358

For Product Safety Concerns and Information please contact
our EU representative GPSR@taylorandfrancis.com Taylor & Francis
Verlag GmbH, Kaufingerstraße 24, 80331 München, Germany

*9 7 8 0 8 6 3 8 8 5 3 5 8 *

T - #0004 - 160425 - C0 - 297/210/12 - SB - 9780863885358 - Gloss Lamination